W9-AVA-372

The Power of
Probiotics
Secrets to Great Health

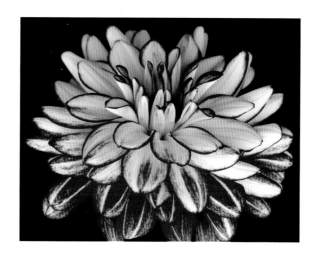

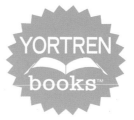

Westlake Village, California USA

Published by Yortren, Inc.

    3180 Willow Lane

    Suite 104

    Westlake Village, CA 91361, USA

Credits:
Book Design: Natasha Trenev, Yordan Trenev
Printer: One World Press, Prescott, AZ
Editor: Carol Crenna
Food Styling: Natasha Trenev, Yordan Trenev, Chef Roberto Carboni, Alice Williams
Food Preparation: Chef Roberto Carboni
Photography: Alice Williams

2

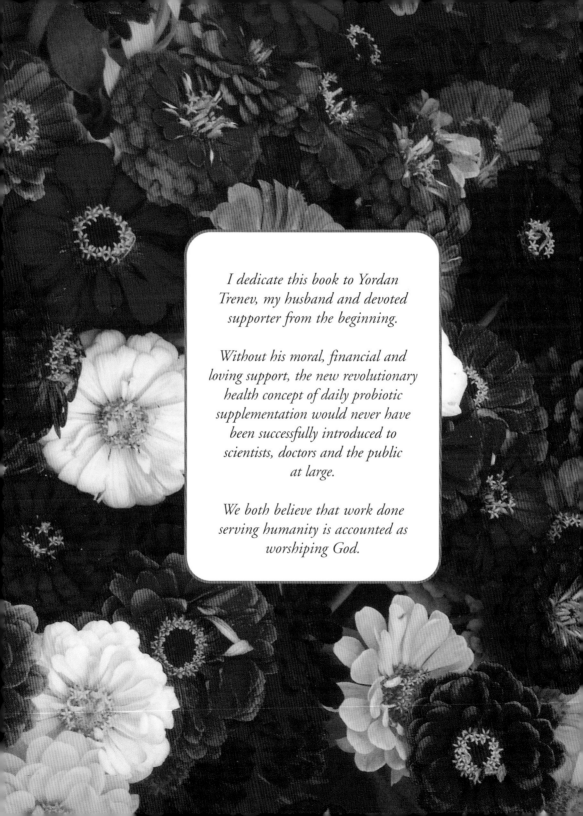

I dedicate this book to Yordan Trenev, my husband and devoted supporter from the beginning.

Without his moral, financial and loving support, the new revolutionary health concept of daily probiotic supplementation would never have been successfully introduced to scientists, doctors and the public at large.

We both believe that work done serving humanity is accounted as worshiping God.

TABLE OF CONTENTS

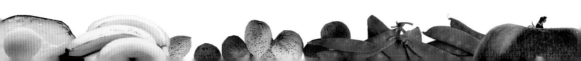

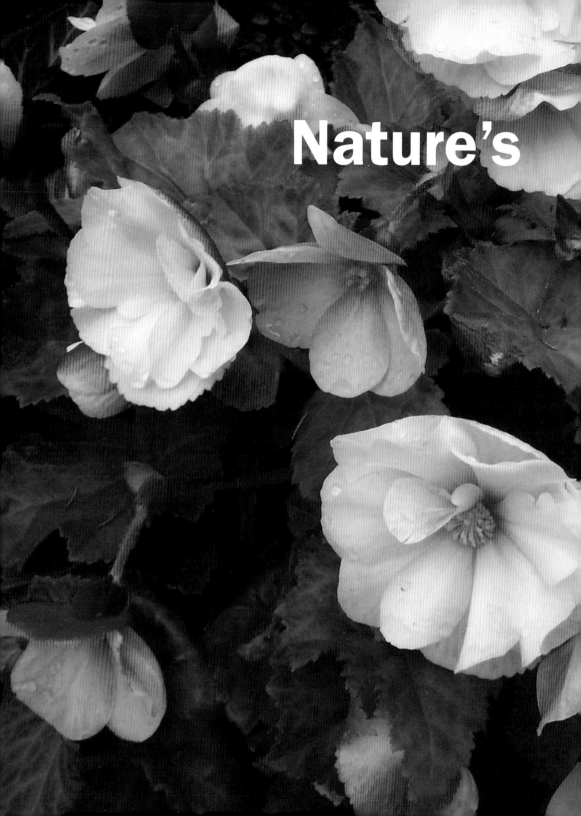

Nature's

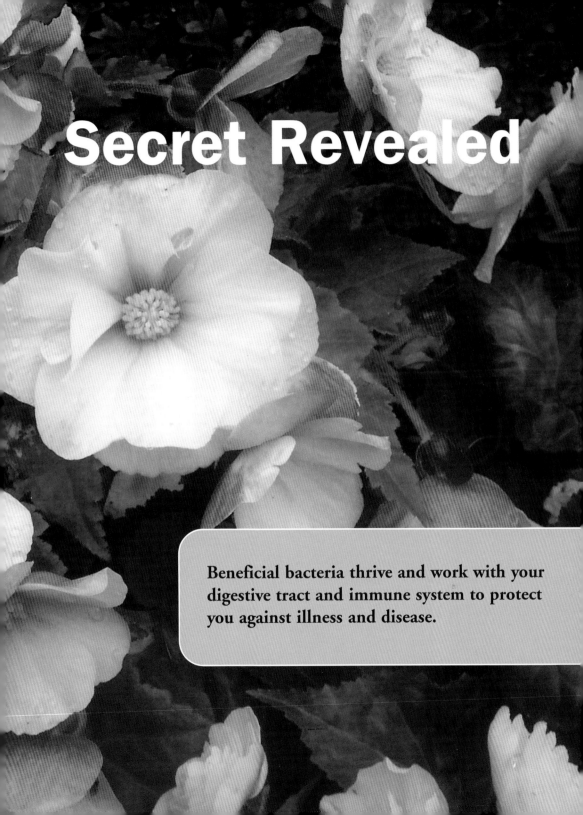

Secret Revealed

Beneficial bacteria thrive and work with your digestive tract and immune system to protect you against illness and disease.

Introduction

Bacteria – In today's world where we battle superbugs, food poisoning and chronic infections, that one simple word can make people cringe. But what would you do if someone told you there were three and a half pounds of bacteria, including *Escherichia coli* (*E. coli*) and salmonella, living inside your intestinal tract right now? Would you take antibiotics to clean out your insides, as you would for a bacterial infection?

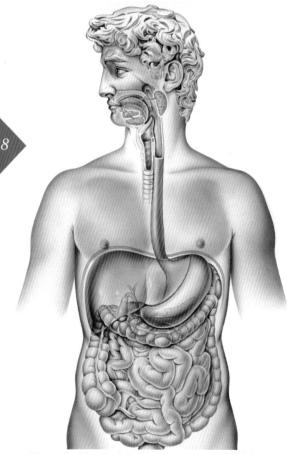

Well, the catch is that if you successfully flush out all of those bacteria, whatever you put in your body next could lead to a life-threatening disease. Do you wonder why this is?

Bacteria are vital to protect you. In fact, those three and a half pounds are a mixture of good, neutral, chameleon and bad bacteria that keep you healthy and alive. These gut microflora (very tiny living organisms) are a major part of your digestive and immune systems. When you are healthy, all of these types of bacteria are in a crucial, very delicate balance. Once your microflora are out of balance, your health is in major jeopardy. In fact, I believe that bacteria, fungi and viruses are the cause of all disorders and diseases.

The gastrointestinal tract is an average of 27 feet in length from mouth to anus.

Stress, pollution, drugs, diet changes, aging, environment and travel, not only to foreign countries but every step you take outside of your home, are all culprits that deplete beneficial bacteria levels, creating an imbalance in your gastrointestinal (digestive system) microflora. Digestive problems, skin conditions, debilitating diseases and even death can result.

Some organisms we encounter daily are not only unfriendly, they are downright dangerous! However, beneficial bacteria help protect you from the onslaught of disease-causing microorganisms. They defend the body against bad bacteria (pathogens including salmonella), detrimental fungi (such as yeast and mold) and viruses (like your annual flu virus).

Micro-miracles we take for granted… Probiotics are good bacteria that help to prevent and even to relieve a variety of health problems including chronic diseases, autoimmune diseases, acid reflux, coronary heart disease, irritable bowel syndrome (IBS), food poisoning and lactose intolerance. I have also found that they alleviate autism and eradicate yeast infections.

Probiotics are defined as "a live microbial feed supplement that beneficially affects the host by improving its intestinal microbial balance." Probiotics, literally meaning "for life," have been known for thousands of years. According to the Food and Agriculture Organization and the World Health Organization, probiotics are "live organisms which, when administered in adequate amounts, confer a health benefit on the host." However, both of these definitions fail to convey the true impact these tiny miracles have on our bodies on a daily basis.

Probiotics – A Brief History

Food serves both as medicine and as nourishment. Revered Greek physician Hippocrates said, "Let food be your medicine and medicine be your food." Throughout history, fermented milk products were used to improve appetite and to treat dysentery, peptic ulcers, diarrhea and other gastric (stomach) disorders.

The usefulness of probiotics was recorded in paintings dating back to 2500 B.C. Sumerians living in the ancient Persian Gulf area had already discovered the cheese making process, which retained milk's dietary appeal. Cultures of lactobacillus, a type of food-fermenting bacteria, transformed milk into cheese and other dairy products. This enabled them to be more easily digested and allowed the milk to remain edible longer.

Ancient Greeks and Romans also produced fermented products using soured milk, honey, flour and fruits. The Emperor of Persia had a special room designated for making yogurt, which was used in human food and for feeding birds and cattle.

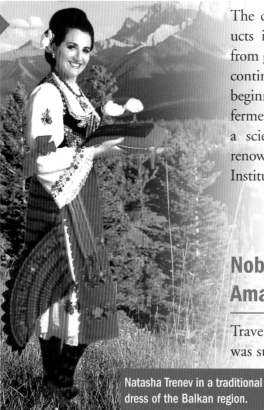

The consumption of these fermented products in many different forms was adopted from generation to generation and, of course, continues today. But, it was not until the beginning of the 1900s that the benefits of fermented milk products were examined from a scientific basis by Elie Metchnikoff, a renowned Russian biologist at the Pasteur Institute in Paris.

Nobel Prize Recipient's Amazing Discovery

Traveling to Eastern Europe, Metchnikoff was surprised to find many Bulgarians were

Natasha Trenev in a traditional dress of the Balkan region.

more than 100 years of age and still enjoying life. Their diet consisted primarily of homegrown vegetables and an abundance of yogurt. Though fresh vegetables probably contributed to their health, Metchnikoff deduced that the most dramatic difference in diet affecting their longevity was the yogurt, so this is where he focused his research. It should also be noted that these centenarians didn't have modern medicine to help recover from illness, so it could be concluded that something in their diet also acted as a powerful illness fighter.

He investigated the benefits of consuming lactic acid bacteria, the family of bacteria (including lactobacillus and bifidobacteria) that flourish in milk. He theorized that these bacteria prevent putrid digestion, which occurs when improperly digested food rots in your gastrointestinal tract (GI). Physicians from eastern cultures have believed for centuries that putrefaction of undigested food may be a major cause of serious diseases.

Metchnikoff observed that many disease-producing organisms died, or failed to develop, in milk containing lactobacillus. Lactobacillus transformed lactose into lactic acid and Metchnikoff confirmed that the acidity generated an environment hostile to pathogenic bacteria. He named the primary yogurt-culturing bacteria *Lactobacillus bulgaricus*, in honor of the Bulgarians.

In another aspect of his research, Metchnikoff formulated the basic theory of how our immune systems fight illness. He discovered that cells called "phagocytes", which are present in every organ, form the body's first line of defense by engulfing bacteria and other disease-causing organisms. He coined the term "phagocytosis" (the eating of cells), which was a highly controversial concept in his day. Metchnikoff and colleague, Paul Ehrlich, were awarded the Nobel Prize in Physiology and Medicine in 1908 for their accomplishment in initiating modern research into immunology.

Metchnikoff was an innovative scientist and his research on immunity was ahead of its time. Prior to him, people did not understand the importance of immunity or how it relates to longevity. He understood how the immune system functions and was able to make the scientific connection linking lactic acid bacteria to improved immunity and, hence, health and longevity.

Pursue Vigorous Longevity Through Beneficial Bacteria

The secret to a long, healthy and vital life is to assist your body in minimizing the growth of harmful (bad) bacteria and encouraging the growth of beneficial (good) bacteria. You should adopt a healthy lifestyle and eat a proper diet in order to nourish your vital intestinal flora. Unfortunately, it is not possible to restore your balanced microflora through proper diet alone. Supplementation with selected strains of probiotic bacteria is necessary. Due to the damage we have done from our inappropriate use of drugs and chemicals, it will take several generations before we will be able to restore the beneficial bacteria naturally to our bodies.

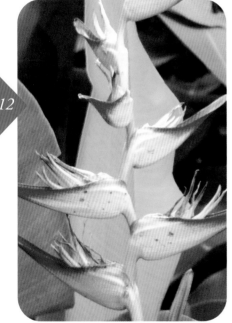

Much like flowers, gastrointestinal microflora will flourish with proper care and replenishment.

Beneficial bacteria are abundant in nature and present on your skin, in your mouth, digestive system and the vaginal mucosa of healthy individuals. Found along with yeast and bad bacteria, they are single-cell organisms occurring biologically alone, in pairs and in short chains. These good bugs perform numerous and indispensable functions to protect you against harmful bacteria, which can cause latent infections that produce chronic illnesses.

Your body needs balance… Beneficial bacteria act as an indispensable defense barrier to repel the attacks mounted by bad bacteria and yeast. When the balance of good and bad bacteria is in harmony, the body operates at its peak. This optimum balance is your guarantee of protection from disease. It is when you lose your optimal balance that trouble begins. The bad bacteria and yeast rapidly spiral out of control, leaving you with a barren intestinal landscape full of toxic waste.

Illness and eventual disease are unavoidable unless you maintain good health with a balanced diet, which includes taking daily probiotic supplements. These beneficial bacteria supplements provide a fast, simple and effective way to promote bowel regularity and elimination of toxins. (More in-depth information on supplements will be given later in this book.) Bowel regularity reduces exposure to many accumulated toxins including harmful substances such as nitrites – a preservative commonly used in meat products.

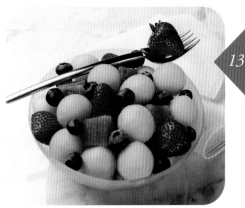

Fresh, healthy foods support the growth of beneficial bacteria.

The most common way to promote regularity is consumption of fiber. However, this may be too harsh for your system because you may already be dealing with inflammation within your intestines, characterized by redness, heat, pain and swelling. Bowel cleansing using harsh products or purging methods, which has become popular in recent years, depletes the beneficial microflora and irritates already inflamed intestinal walls.

I strongly advise against bowel cleansing in this unnatural way. It will adversely alter the balance of the 100 trillion bacteria that reside in the GI tract, leaving the body vulnerable to pathogens that can take control. Because seventy percent of the immune system is located in the GI tract, this disruption of the flora not only reduces the absorption of essential nutrients, it has a dramatically negative effect on immunity. If you use one of these cleansing products you may not be aware of the side effects until they surface weeks or even years later.

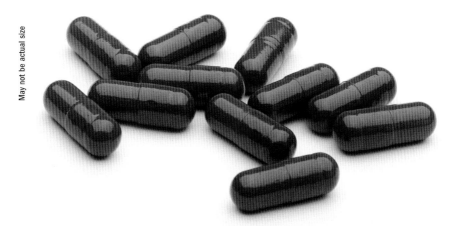

May not be actual size

Supplements made from selected strains of lactobacillus and bifidobacteria are safe and non-toxic at any level.

Going "pro"... Probiotic supplements that combine "validated" (meaning a neutral authoritative body has audited the claims) selected strains of beneficial bacteria offer the safest, most effective solution. These carefully selected, stringently tested probiotics maintain healthy intestinal flora that are necessary to keep dangerous bacteria in check. Not only do they control the growth of bad bacteria and reduce the toxic load of harmful byproducts from normal body metabolism, chemicals in food and in the environment, they minimize the inflammatory cycle and allow the intestinal wall to heal. These valuable health promoters perform indispensable functions that help the body tolerate lactose (the sugar found in dairy products that is difficult to digest), keep the vaginal tract healthy and inhibit opportunistic, disease-causing pathogens. They boost the immune system and stimulate the body's tolerance to food and environmental elements. They help you avoid allergic reactions and optimize the absorption of essential vitamins and minerals from food and dietary supplements.

Become supplement savvy… Be aware that all supplements containing beneficial bacteria are not created equal. Selected super strains of bacteria that are derived from human origin are the only choice to obtain the many benefits of probiotics. Validated super strains yield the most effective natural substances for protecting the intestines from harmful bacteria. Be sure to do your research before buying and then check the bottle's label listing these bacteria, since proper strain selection is your assurance of reliable quality. Other strains have been proven to be weaker and less effective for humans. Powerful super strains, used in researched products, include the following:

Lactobacillus acidophilus is the most prominent resident bacteria in the small intestine. Super strains called NAS and DDS-1 have demonstrated increased production of hydrogen peroxide (H_2O_2), which destroys bad bacteria, yeast and viruses, and have proven antimicrobial and antifungal characteristics.*

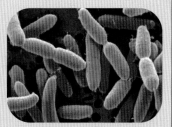

Bifidobacterium bifidum is the powerful supporter of the large intestine, regulating unwanted bacterial growth and acting as your all-important waste and disposal system. Super strain Malyoth is the most potent and beneficial strain of resident bifidobacterium available. It has been validated in clinical trials with cirrhotic liver patients as an important support system to repair damaged livers.*

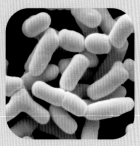

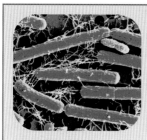

Lactobacillus bulgaricus is the transient bacteria supporting a healthy GI tract by helping to digest complex carbohydrates and proteins. Super strain LB-51 increases the absorption of essential minerals (especially calcium) while supporting the helpful action of *Lactobacillus acidophilus* and *Bifidobacterium bifidum*.*

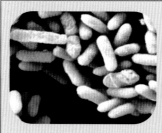

Bifidobacterium infantis is the most important bacteria for the development of a healthy infant, minimizing the predisposition to allergies and encouraging the production of antibodies. Super strain NLS is the essential "baby bacteria", which stimulates better weight gain and assists in the absorption of nutrients and vitamins.*

These images represent the species of bacteria but not the unique super strains.

16

Preferences for using certain probiotic strains vary by geographical region based on diet, with lactobacillus, especially *Lactobacillus acidophilus*, holding higher regard in the western part of the world and bifidobacteria commanding greater respect in areas along the Pacific Rim. However, both types are fundamental to your health. Beneficial bacteria are not found or used in isolation within the body. They work together to promote health. They also do not function in isolation in only one part of the body. They are found in many organs and systems.

When you open a bottle of supplements, you don't always know what's inside... You don't really know if the ingredients are active (and therefore potent) and, even more important, whether they are disruptive, offsetting your body's delicate balance. It is critical, therefore, that the strains you select have been proven safe. Both *Lactobacillus* and *Bifidobacterium* genera (families) have extensive proven track records in safety through centuries of use in fermented foods. (Please refer to the purchasing probiotics section in this book for more information.) A poor product offers no assurance of success. Only buy products from a manufacturer you can trust – a company that offers validated super strains with guaranteed potency and that provides a clearly printed expiration date on the bottle. Many products on the market are misbranded and do not contain what is listed on the label. I will help you to make the right choices by giving you "TOP TIPS" on finding selected powerful, health-promoting probiotics.

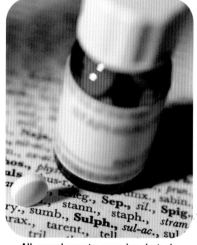

All supplements promise but do they deliver?

Top Tip: *Lactobacillus acidophilus* was first isolated and classified in 1900, following the isolation of *Lactobacillus bifidus*. Later research proved *bifidus* was inaccurately grouped in the *Lactobacillus* genus, having significant differences in structure and nutritional requirements. In 1974, the organisms were designated as a separate genus, *Bifidobacterium*. Beware of manufacturers that use *Lactobacillus bifidus* or *L. bifidus* on a label as this is incorrect terminology and shows that they do not know exactly what they are selling.

The bold strength of bifido… Bifidobacteria include more than a dozen species and hundreds of strains. Professor Tomotari Mitsuoka of the University of Tokyo, Department of Biomedical Science has researched this type of bacteria's vital function to the host's (your) health and prospects for longevity. He reports, "It is now clear that bifidobacteria … are far more important than *Lactobacillus acidophilus* as beneficial intestinal bacteria, throughout human life."

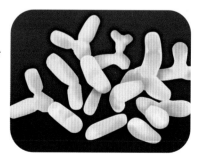

Bifid-o-bacteria were named after their 'Y' shape.

Lactobacillus bulgaricus is found in traditional Bulgarian-style yogurt. Researchers inspired by Metchnikoff's findings decided to follow up on his theories in the 1950s. Dr. Ivan Bogdanov of Bulgaria and his colleagues isolated a unique strain of *Lactobacillus bulgaricus* and identified it as LB-51. For the first time, they established that LB-51 produces a natural antibiotic substance that has a wide spectrum of antibacterial activity, proving that the long-living Bulgarians were eating a potent illness fighter.

Reinforcing Your Internal Army – How Probiotics Work

Ideally, a person in optimal health should have billions of bifidobacteria and lactobacillus, including *Lactobacillus acidophilus* and *Lactobacillus bulgaricus*, marching out to defend them. Unfortunately, many environmental factors affect your overall health and leave you in a less than optimal state.

Causes of Bacterial Depletion		
• Pollution	• Diet	• Traveling
• Aging	• Drugs	• Radiation
• Illness	• Chemotherapy	• Eating Disorders
• Colonics	• Cesarean Delivery	• Infants Born in
• Formula Feeding	• Environmental	Westernized
• Stress	Changes	Urban Areas

When natural defenses are depleted, you are left with a barren intestinal landscape that can be easily and rapidly colonized by pathogens or harmful yeast (more on yeast provided later). You are also left with a weakened immune system that is unable to fight disease and infection. This is why you must constantly replenish internal protectors to maintain your first line of defense.

Selected strains of probiotic supplements boost your body's beneficial bacteria, rebuilding your natural defenses by functioning in four ways:

1) Probiotics produce substances that stop the growth of pathogenic bacteria and harmful yeast. The substances include lactic acid, the primary byproduct, as well as bacteriocins, antibiotics, and antimicrobial and antifungal compounds.
2) Probiotics have metabolic activities that physiologically benefit the host (the person they live inside). This could include improved lactose tolerance, reduced toxins produced by other intestinal microbes and improved sugar, carbohydrate and protein digestion.
3) Probiotics compete with other organisms in the body for nutrients and adhesion sites, thereby displacing or blocking the adhesion of harmful microorganisms.
4) Probiotics stimulate the immune system to fight infectious agents causing inflammation. They also reduce incidences of an over-reacting immune system (which can cause everything from allergies to debilitating autoimmune disorders) by calming the hyper-allergenic response and inflammatory cycles throughout the body.

These benefits, however, are species and strain specific. Only validated beneficial bacteria strains deliver them.

A barren intestinal landscape cannot protect you from disease-causing bacteria or yeast.

Don't be misled. Learn how to distinguish which probiotics are the right ones to choose.

Numerous public studies have revealed the continuous failure of products to meet their label declarations. Among them were tests by Bastyr University, Consumer Labs and *Consumer Reports*.

Shelf sampling of twenty lactobacillus supplements by researchers from Bastyr University revealed that none of the brands tested had organisms identical to the ones listed on their label. Half of the products contained microorganisms not listed on the label. Six included an organism that could cause illness or pass along antibiotic resistance.

Consumer Labs tested twenty-five probiotic products and found alarming results. Six products had only a few thousand live bacteria; products that low in bacterial count would have little effectiveness. In the study, thirteen of the products claimed specific numbers of live organisms only at the time of manufacture, not indicating the number that would be in the product at the time of use.

A study published in *Consumer Reports* from independent laboratories tested fourteen probiotic supplements. They found that most brands list bacterial count at time of manufacture. Testing revealed four of the fourteen had less than half the count listed. These guarantees at time of manufacture are misleading to the unaware consumer.

Consumer Labs stated that "neither the FDA nor any other federal or state agency routinely test probiotics for quality prior to sale." However, other countries have stringent regulations for dietary supplements. In an unprecedented action, the government of Australia recalled more than 1,600 products. Among those products were several probiotic supplements. However, the products by a brand called Natren, which are validated by third-party auditors, were not recalled.

Live Healthy and Happy – Probiotic Health Benefits

The four probiotics functions listed previously are actually only broad categories of the numerous benefits of probiotics as a whole. The following is a more in-depth look at the ways selected strains of probiotics can benefit you.

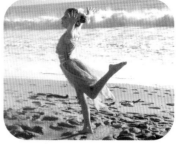

Beneficial bacteria empower you to obtain optimal health.

Health Effects of Selected Strains of Probiotic Bacteria

1) Increased nutritional value through better digestibility and increased absorption of minerals and vitamins
2) Normalization of gut function, relieving constipation and irritable bowel syndrome
3) Reduction in urinary and vaginal tract infections caused by bacteria and yeast
4) Inhibition of *Helicobacter pylori*, the bacterial cause of stomach ulcers
5) Prevention of GI tract infections caused by bacteria, viruses or yeast
6) Improvement of kidney and liver function by elimination of toxins
7) Repopulation of beneficial flora following antibiotics or radiation
8) Reduction of the hyper-allergenic reactions of the immune system
9) Improved well-being and optimal physical and mental health
10) Prevention of atherosclerosis by reducing blood cholesterol
11) Stimulation of the immune system to boost defenses
12) Increased resistance to infectious disease
13) Reduction of disease-inducing agents
14) Improvement of lactose digestion
15) Decreased duration of diarrhea
16) Reduction in blood pressure
17) Prevention of osteoporosis
18) Reduction of allergies

When good goes bad... It's important to note that even good bacteria that exhibit indispensable properties (like those previously listed) in laboratory tests may not retain their ability to function optimally when in a supplement. This is due to the fact that when they are manufactured, there may be variations from batch to batch unless their stability is maintained throughout production. Optimal stability is similar to mass-producing a superb cake a thousand times without losing any of its delicious features. It is crucial to select products from a respected manufacturer that has the skill, experience and knowledge to consistently produce an effective probiotic product.

There are several critical factors involved in producing beneficial bacteria supplements that will enable you to obtain the best possible health benefits. The manufacturer must incorporate the following standards into the production process:

- Strain selection – choose and grow the best bacteria;
- Growth medium – use a culturing base that enables the bacteria to express their specialized benefits, such as antimicrobial substances;
- Production and stabilization procedures – train the bacteria to develop their specific benefits in support of your health.

I feel that it is vital to look to a manufacturer who specializes in validated, single strain probiotic bacteria products. A single strain has a unique genetic makeup that makes it superior. It has a strongly proven track record for imparting specialized health benefits. Choose one that provides a meaningful guarantee of potency and strain specificity through an expiration date printed on the label.

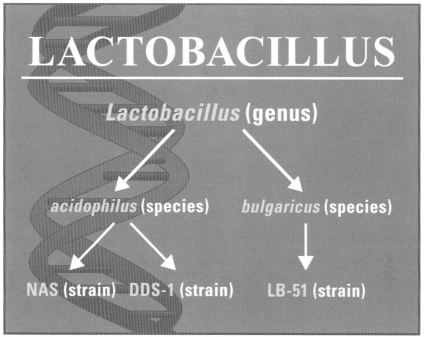

LACTOBACILLUS

Lactobacillus (genus)

acidophilus **(species)**   *bulgaricus* **(species)**

NAS (strain)   DDS-1 (strain)   LB-51 (strain)

Bacteria family tree

Probiotics include many genera and species, and each species includes hundreds of strains of bacteria. Each unique strain has its own specialized roles and benefits that are passed on to you, the host. For example, when strains of lactobacillus are fermented, they produce antimicrobial substances, which kill bacteria and other microorganisms. These substances include lactic acid, acetic acid, formic acid and hydrogen peroxide (H_2O_2). The hydrogen peroxide produced from *Lactobacillus acidophilus*, NAS and DDS-1 super strains is a natural and very potent antibacterial, antifungal and antiviral compound. This hydrogen peroxide production is a proven feature of these two super strains.

Lactobacillus acidophilus, DDS-1 super strain produces the antimicrobial substance acidophilin, which is active against a wide spectrum of bacteria, yeasts and fungi. *Lactobacillus acidophilus*, DDS-1 super strain is only capable of producing acidophilin when it is "over-cultured",

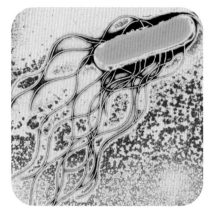

The salmonella bacteria are a leading cause of food poisoning, gastric illness and chronic autoimmune disease.

grown and fermented longer than normal, in milk. Acidophilin has a powerfully inhibiting effect on bad bacteria including *Clostridium botulinum,* salmonella bacteria, *Staphylococcus aureus* and *Escherichia coli* (*E. coli*) – major culprits in food poisoning and intestinal disease. *Bifidobacterium bifidum,* Malyoth super strain and *Lactobacillus bulgaricus,* LB-51 super strain also act to suppress these and other injurious bacteria and fungi. These two super strains defeat pathogens by producing their own specialized antimicrobial compounds.

Top Tip: Be wary of fake DDS-1 cultures. Only one manufacturer, Natren, has independent validation that it has had DDS-1 strain in its products since 1982.

A bug's life… All bacteria are intelligent living organisms that engage in complex behavior. This cannot be explained or fully appreciated simply by discussing their single benefits or actions. These beneficial bacteria communicate with each other biochemically or by using photon light emissions. They do this with special cells including epithelial cells (cells that cover your body organs), macrophages (scavenger cells that fight disease), T-cells (the most powerful disease-killing cells) and other components of the immune system. When necessary, many beneficial strains, such as the ones listed above, can calm down over-reactive inflammatory responses while they stimulate the immune system for optimal protection.

Billions of microbial interactions take place continuously throughout the GI tract. These interactions can be compromised or improved depending on environmental, physiological and emotional changes.

By continuously supplementing with the proper beneficial bacteria you will have the best insurance to maintain a stable, balanced and optimally healthy GI tract.

Bacterial Balancing Act – How Good and Bad Coexist

The GI tract's microflora are made up of good, bad and neutral bacteria, which are the smallest of living organisms. The good bacteria are known as beneficial bacteria because they help keep potentially harmful bacteria from becoming established. Beneficial bacteria also have the ability to manufacture vitamins and natural antibiotics, as well as communicate with the immune system to minimize allergies or stimulate rapid response to an invasion by disease-causing microorganisms. Bad bacteria are known as pathogens and they can make you sick, cause disease and threaten your life. Neutral bacteria and

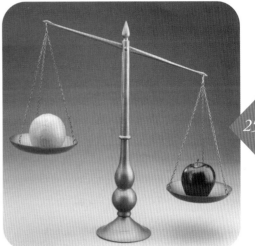

A proper and essential balance of intestinal microflora is needed for great health.

yeast, also known as chameleons because they can disguise themselves and hide from the immune system, become harmful under certain conditions (e.g., after antibiotic therapy or when the immune system is compromised).

Overwhelming scientific evidence supports the importance of beneficial bacteria to human health and longevity. As long as the body's immune system remains strong, resident pathogens keep a low profile.

This is probably the most studied natural phenomenon in the scientific community.

Your body has transient (traveling) good bacteria, as well as resident good bacteria, with "adhesive" properties, which increase their ability to adhere to the intestinal wall. But even bacteria with superior adhesive properties may get scraped off the intestinal wall by competitive bacteria, a high fiber diet, stress, pollution and the natural process of new cells replacing old cells on the intestinal lining.

Transient bacteria do not set up colonies inside of our GI tract but they do provide help while traveling through. They help resident bacteria grow, which, in turn, keeps the bad bacteria from flourishing. *Lactobacillus bulgaricus* and *Streptococcus thermophilus* are the best-known and most effective transient bacteria recognized worldwide as the two symbiotic bacteria (mutually benefiting each other through their interactions) used to produce yogurt.

Daily life, global pollution of natural resources and abuse of antibiotics reduce your natural levels of beneficial bacteria dramatically. Harmful bacteria are entering your body, and everyone else's, in larger numbers more than ever before in history. The increased numbers of bad bacteria initiate a hostile takeover of your GI tract by the resident pathogens living within you. Selected probiotic bacteria strains increase your

Pollution is one of the factors causing depleted levels of beneficial bacteria.

numbers of beneficial bacteria, which flourish and strengthen your first line of defense against pathogenic invasions.

To fully understand the benefits of probiotic bacteria, you must have a clear understanding of what happens within your body's GI tract.

Battle of the Bugs – Competition for Dominance in the GI Tract

There are approximately 1,000 different species of microorganisms teeming within the body's intestinal tract. Your body houses 100 trillion microorganisms – more than ten times the number of cells in your body – and they are all competing for territorial dominance.

The invaluable GI tract, which begins at the mouth and ends at the anus, is the ultimate arbitrator of both health and disease. Approximately twenty-seven feet long (depending on your height), the GI tract is a fueling station, helping to nourish and improve immune function, and provide your body with a vital continuous nutrient supply. It is also a waste-management system and a waste-disposal system. Probiotic strains are essential in neutralizing toxic byproducts not removed through bowel elimination. The whole purpose of digestion is to extract every bit of nourishment from food and continuously expel what the body does not need.

Food and water consumed on a daily basis contain large amounts of harmful microorganisms, most of which are excreted as dry-weight fecal matter. The stomach contains only a trace amount, if any, of these microorganisms, due to its formidable acid barrier that minimizes their survival. It is important to maintain that acid barrier in your stomach to promote a healthy, protective environment in the digestive tract.

If you are in optimal health, you have a protective barrier of beneficial bacteria adhering to the epithelial cells on the wall of the GI tract. The normal flora repel the invasive army of pathogens waiting to establish territorial dominance. When this protective barrier of beneficial bacteria is reduced due to life events (such as poor eating habits, infection, antibiotics, injury and stress), the pathogens' wait is over. Stimulated by the opportunity for nutrients, they multiply and damage the epithelial cells. Toxins produced by the pathogens cause more damage, destroying the tight junctions between the cells of the intestinal wall. Now they have access to the bloodstream and a free ride to infect organs in remote locations in the body.

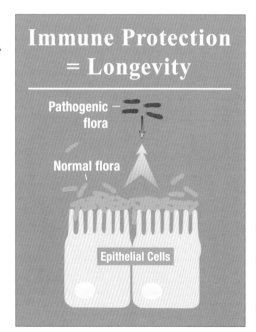

Immune Protection = Longevity

Pathogenic flora

Normal flora

Epithelial Cells

Beneficial bacteria defend the epithelial cells.

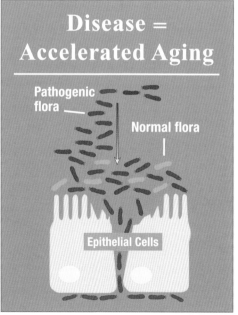

Disease = Accelerated Aging

Pathogenic flora

Normal flora

Epithelial Cells

Pathogens attack and damage the epithelial cells.

Evolution of Harmful Bacteria – Single Cells With a Brain

According to the World Health Organization, chronic disease will kill 400 million people by 2015, but many of those deaths can be prevented by healthier lifestyles and inexpensive medications.

The primary causes of today's slow-burning plagues are parasites, viruses, bacteria and infectious microbes, according to Dr. Paul Ewald, professor of Biology at Amherst College. He conceived the new medical discipline called "evolutionary medicine." He observed that invading microbes, which take up long-term residence in your body, evolve very rapidly. His research found that evolutionary changes in antibiotic resistance occur in just a few weeks. The invading pathogens that cause harmful infections are incredibly clever, either hiding in your cells to avoid detection by the immune system or disguising themselves to resemble human tissues. By doing so, they go unrecognized by your body's defense army.

Dr. Ewald explains that a certain germ can actually disguise itself as a heart cell and if it does, the immune system targeting the foreign germ will attack the heart as well. One innovative bacterium, *Bacteroides fragilis*, hijacks a cloak of fucose, a simple sugar, from the surface of the epithelial cells to cover itself. This confuses the body and gives the pathogens the time they need to proliferate into large numbers. Tragically, while the pathogen is reproducing, the immune system is busy mounting a defense that will attack the mimicked human cells as well as the body's own tissue.

Fungi: Lying in wait... *Candida albicans* is another such resourceful, resident pathogen. Candida is a member of the fungi family and can exist in two forms, as a yeast bud in a single-cell organism and as a mold. It can rapidly transform from a chameleon yeast to a looming threat in the mold form. Normally, yeast comprises ten

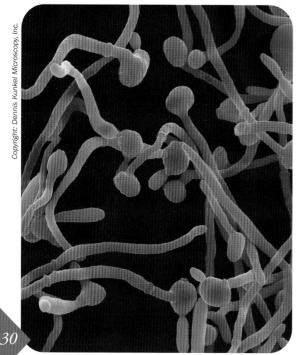

Candida albicans – Neutral yeast buds and pathogenic cross-branching mold structure.

percent of the microorganisms in our intestinal tract. When the delicate balance of beneficial bacteria is upset, the yeast proliferates rapidly. This aggressive and uncontrolled growth allows the yeast to transform into pathogenic mold, a cross-branching formation that can attach and pierce the soft tissues of the body, triggering a host of symptoms and health problems.

The medical community has underestimated the threat that *Candida albicans* poses. Unfortunately, since they don't take it seriously, there is considerable confusion because most people think of it as simple nail fungus or vaginal irritation. Among natural health practitioners, there is an opposing view that candida alone is the cause of multiple ailments. I feel that these are both overly simplified points of view that do not consider the complexity of the microbial world.

Candida works in harmony with other bacteria and viruses to compromise your health. Just as bacteria become resistant to drugs, and viruses mutate to avoid being killed off, candida becomes resistant to antifungal drugs. No treatment can target and kill all of the microorganisms involved in a disease. Your inner world of microbiology does not tolerate a void. Unless you repopulate it with selected super strains of probiotics, you cannot control the microorganisms that re-grow to fill that void or their negative effect on your health.

Another chameleon microorganism is *Bacillus cereus*, one of many types of soil bacteria that can adopt any DNA it comes in contact with. *Bacillus cereus* causes two types of food-borne illness: one characterized by vomiting and the other causing diarrhea, abdominal cramps and nausea. Although *Bacillus cereus* was not considered to be life threatening in the past, more recent reports have linked a strain that produces increased amounts of toxin to death caused by liver failure. Note that *Bacillus cereus* can form spores capable of surviving heat (and cooking) for a prolonged period, and is difficult to kill.

Many soil organisms are misidentified and inappropriately used in probiotic products for human consumption. When used indiscriminately in an unregulated probiotic supplement, I stress that these soil organisms will pose unknown and possibly serious dangers to human beings because they can change shapes. This can cause serious diseases. (This will be explained in a later book in this series.)

The good, the bad and the ugly…

Bacteria have a perverse ability to change their nature as they evolve. The once-mellow family of bacteria called enterococcus was fairly insignificant prior to the growing problem of antibiotic

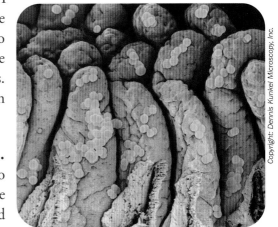

Copyright: Dennis Kunkel Microscopy, Inc.

Staphylococcus aureus is the number one cause of two million hospital-borne infections each year.

overuse. The stomach and GI tract held billions of these enterococci, but they were so inoffensive that 10,000 times as many enterococci as *Staphylococcus aureus* bacteria were required to kill a person. *Staphylococcus aureus*, a deadly pathogen, is the number one cause of an estimated 2 million hospital-borne infections in the U.S. each year. The evolutionary ecological shift has prompted enterococci to become a more perilous threat.

> **Top tip:** Never buy probiotic supplements containing *Enterococcus faecium* (*E. faecium*) or *Enterococcus faecalis* (*E. faecalis*). Previously known as streptococcus, these two microbes are a medical menace. Both microbes developed resistance to vancomycin, an extremely powerful drug and one of the few antibiotics that could reliably kill staph bacteria that cause fatal infections. Vancomycin resistance jumped from *Enterococcus faecium* and *Enterococcus faecalis* to *Staphylococcus aureus*, and so the dreaded flesh-eating super bug gained extraordinary power to infect people while repelling vancomycin treatment.

As antibiotic use became popular, the beneficial bacteria receded, leaving a wide-open invitation for the very opportunistic enterococci to spread. Throughout a thirty-year period, enterococci were routinely exposed to vancomycin, the antibiotic used against *Staphylococcus aureus*. Without attracting much attention, enterococci gradually developed resistance and eventually succeeded in generating a vancomycin-resistant gene. Vancomycin is known as the drug of last resort and is commonly used to treat patients with severe infections. The mighty enterococci are the leaders of all microorganisms in teaching other microbes to develop resistance to new drugs.

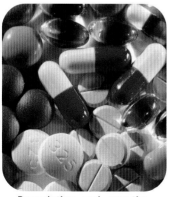

Prescription and over-the-counter drugs deplete beneficial bacteria levels.

Unfortunately, modern medicine's traditional approach to chronic problems – antibiotics, prescription and nonprescription drugs – kills bacteria, pathogens and beneficial bacteria alike. The disastrous result of this is an environment left unguarded by beneficial bacteria and wide open for colonization by fungi, including yeasts and mold, **which antibiotics cannot kill**. Fungal overgrowth, a health problem of major proportion, then takes over and renders a toxic or imbalanced GI tract, a possible breeding ground for problems such as mental illness, heart disease and other serious afflictions.

The solution to modern medicine's detrimental approach and the pathogens' increasing ability to adjust can be found in a system of daily probiotic supplementation. Probiotics are the missing link to optimal wellness – *truly the foundation of your good health*. Beneficial bacteria form colonies that reside on the intestinal wall in your GI tract to defend against the potentially harmful microorganisms you inhale from the air and ingest from food and water.

The GI microflora are dynamic – changing daily in relation to your genetic predisposition, lifestyle, diet, stress level, mental outlook and travel. Unhealthy organisms are continually trying to gain dominance on your skin and in your body. Science validates the need to replenish the body's probiotic forces daily, with clinical studies proving that adding certain good bacteria helps replace what has been lost and helps to strengthen the army of good against bad to face daily obstacles. Supplementing with a validated selected strain of probiotic bacteria should become a ritual … as routine as brushing your teeth.

Top Tip: Do not buy an inferior product, because it won't deliver the same health benefits, wasting your time and money. Check whether the manufacturer is licensed under International Drug Good Manufacturing Practice (GMP) to ensure the product you are purchasing is potent, pure and safe.

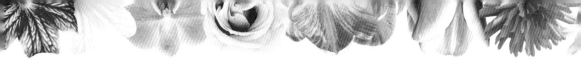

The Birth of Good Bugs – How Your Microflora Is Established

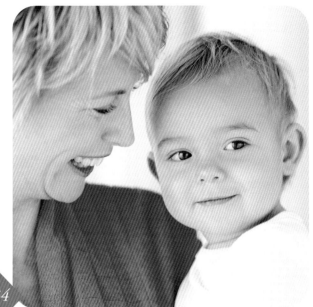

A mother's health while pregnant and nursing continuously determines the levels of beneficial microflora in her infant's gut.

34

Your mother's health plays a significant role in the amount and selection of beneficial bacteria you acquire at birth. You obtain your initial dose of beneficial bacteria as you pass through the birth canal. If you were delivered in a hospital, any harmful and drug-resistant bacteria inhabiting the hospital room will also affect your health. These initial bacteria will influence your overall well-being and future immunity to allergies and chronic infections. The bacteria determine how efficiently your body digests food and absorbs nutrients, and whether you can thrive as an infant to grow strong and beat health challenges.

Infants delivered vaginally by mothers in good health are bathed with friendly, protective bifidobacteria as they pass through the birth canal. These beneficial bacteria establish attachment sites on the GI wall, forming a protective flora before not-so-friendly microorganisms attempt to dominate the body. Infants born via a cesarean section do not receive this bath of beneficial bacteria.

Build baby's defense through breast-feeding... Breast-feeding is the second step to helping your child's intestinal microflora flourish.

When infants are breast-fed by healthy mothers, protective microflora comprised almost entirely of bifidobacteria are established. This process stimulates intestinal peristalsis, the wave-like contraction of the small intestines that keeps food moving steadily through the digestive tract. More importantly, this helps infants have acidic stools (pH 5.0-5.5), which inhibit the growth of disease-causing bacteria.

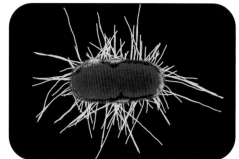

Some strains of *Escherichia coli*, such as *E. coli* O157:H7, cause severe diarrhea, gastrointestinal illness and kidney failure.

Breast-feeding protects your newborn against infectious disease. This protection is a result of the hundreds of different potent nutrients and components unique to human breast milk that stimulate the infant's immune system. Breast milk contains antimicrobial compounds and numerous growth factors that help stabilize the immature gut and decrease the risk of intestinal disturbances from diarrhea-causing bacteria, such as *Escherichia coli* (*E. coli*) and *Vibrio cholera*.

Dr. Michael L. McCann, M.D., FAAP, states, "A cesarean section infant who is fed cows' milk formula or receives antibiotics is in double jeopardy." This is due to the lack of beneficial bacteria following birth as well as a continued lack of receiving beneficial bacteria through breast milk. Human breast milk contains over 100 different beneficial constituents that aren't found in cow's milk. Cow's milk makeup is very different since it is naturally meant to nourish a very quickly growing calf with four stomachs. With far more protein and far less carbohydrates than found in human breast milk, cow's milk is very difficult for a human to digest. Lacking the beneficial bacteria found in human milk can lead to indigestion and leaky gut beginning as early as infancy.

The proper digestion of your infant's food (just like your food) depends on his or her gut microflora. Beneficial bacteria break down large complex proteins into small components that are easily digested by their immature gut. When the gut microflora are unbalanced the gut walls become leaky. Large undigested food proteins can pass through the gut walls and enter the bloodstream. The invasion of these large proteins triggers an allergic reaction. The immune system then memorizes the inflammatory response caused by the allergic reaction and is conditioned to over-react every time it is exposed to those foods. I have found, and research has proven my position, that selected strains of probiotic bacteria calm the immune system so that normal food proteins can be tolerated and the allergic reaction is reduced.

Is Breast-Feeding Enough? – Supplements for Good Beginnings

Your newborn's defenses are not fully formed and not experienced – they're like a newly trained army that knows little about its enemies and how to fight them. In newborns, the previously sterile GI tract rapidly acquires bacteria from the birth process as well as surrounding environment. After birth, infants are continuously exposed to new microbes that enter the GI tract with food. In breast-fed infants, the bacteria originate from the nipple and surrounding skin as well as the milk ducts in the breast. *Bifidobacterium* species are the predominant organisms in the

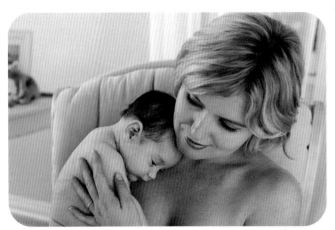
Breast-feeding is the natural way for a mother to pass on beneficial bacteria to her infant.

large intestine of breast-fed infants, accounting for about ninety-nine percent of the flora. More specifically, *Bifidobacterium infantis* is the dominant organism in the gut microflora of infants fortunate enough to get them from a healthy mother who also has the right species of bacteria (see below).

The health of your child's defense system starts with the foods you eat... While pregnant, the nutrients in your foods and supplements nourish the unborn fetus and your immune system protects your unborn infant from infections that may threaten you. After birth, your infant is no longer protected by your body from harmful elements. The gut microflora are relatively unstable and may be easily upset by small changes in your diet or common infections that you can easily fight off. Even a change in your emotional state can affect the quality of breast milk. Therefore, the strength of your infant's future immunity depends on you – your diet, your emotions and your state of health. This is primarily influenced by the composition of your GI microflora. This is why it is important to boost your immune system by taking selected strains of probiotics throughout your pregnancy and daily while breast-feeding.

A twenty-year study conducted in Germany (1958-1977) saw a decline in the number of good bifidobacteria in breast-fed infants and an increase in the presence of bad, pathogenic bacteria, such as *Escherichia coli* (*E. coli*), Klebsiella and Proteus. The champion baby bacteria, *Bifidobacterium infantis,* disappeared due to changes in that country's lifestyle and environment. This change proved to be a monumental environmental disaster for infants in the western world.

Further research on microflora found that only twenty percent of sixty-one breast-fed infants in a University of Pennsylvania hospital study had a significant number of bifidobacteria. And just two-thirds of twenty-one breast-fed infants in a suburban hospital study had significant numbers of bifidobacteria. These studies further demonstrate that breast-feeding alone, particularly in urban areas, is not sufficient for infants' optimal well-being.

Another study showed that infants from Ghana had high levels of the good bacteria, *Bifidobacterium infantis*, while infants from the United Kingdom and New Zealand had none of the bacteria. As a result, infants in Ghana experienced lower incidences of atopic diseases (a certain type of allergic reaction), such as asthma, eczema and allergic rhinitis (nasal inflammation). In contrast, occurrence of atopic diseases was high among infants from the United Kingdom and New Zealand. The researchers found that the presence of *Bifidobacterium infantis* helps calm the allergic inflammatory responses triggered by the immature immune system. This bacteria helps infants to develop, resulting in a stronger, more tolerant immune system, which means fewer allergies throughout their life.

I know that these are alarming findings considering that Ghana is thought to be a third world country and yet its infants are healthier than ours in some respects. This is a consequence of our increasing environmental contamination including air, water and food pollution, radioactive substances, antibiotics, pesticides and toxic compounds. These contaminants get passed on unnoticed from mother to child.

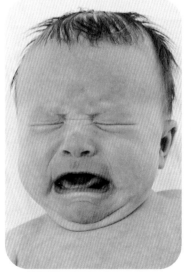

Indigestion can affect and hurt infants too.

When the already fragile bacterial balance in the infant's immature GI tract is disturbed, some infants may not digest food properly. These "fussy" infants are often diagnosed with colic, which is an affliction linked to gastrointestinal distress. Infants who receive high amounts of beneficial bacteria early on and throughout the developing process have lower incidences of colic. Again, these bacteria are usually received through healthy breast milk (unpolluted by the environment) and supplementation of the correct baby-beneficial bacteria – *Bifidobacterium infantis.*

Remember, not all bacteria are created equal and not all bacteria are suitable for an infant's developing system. I strongly advise supplementing with *Bifidobacterium infantis,* NLS super strain on a daily basis, even for breast-fed infants, to encourage the proper balance of bacteria for optimal GI health throughout their life. As a health researcher, I was the first to stress the importance of supplementing with the *Bifidobacterium infantis* species to improve infant health as early as 1984. I introduced the first pure *Bifidobacterium infantis,* NLS super strain for infant use in North America. I know of no company in the world, except for Natren, selling products containing pure *Bifidobacterium infantis,* NLS super strain bacteria for infant use.

Top Tip: All probiotics do not deliver these specific health benefits. Some probiotic supplements use bacteria that are hardy and can be cultured easily and inexpensively. However, these products do not deliver superior and specific health benefits.

Continued Depletion – Modern Medicine Is Not Helping

Your infant's health is highly influenced by what you put into their developing body, even when they're ill and need treatment. Antibiotics have long been thought to be the magical cure-all for any ailment. However, researchers are now finding something quite different. One U.S. study found that infants given antibiotics during the first six months of their lives are far more likely to develop asthma.

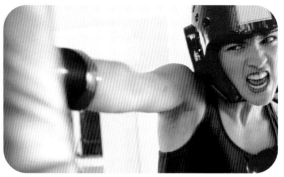

Antibiotics given to infants knock out their fragile, developing microflora.

"Throwing the baby out with the bath water": Antibiotics kill good and bad... Antibiotics are routinely given to infants for numerous ailments, including ear infections and diarrhea. It has been found that two out of three infants have had antibiotics by their first birthday and the figures jump up to three out of four infants receiving antibiotics by their second birthday. This vast overuse and misuse is astounding. Antibiotics do not just kill the bad bacteria causing the infection. They kill indiscriminately. Good bacteria are annihilated as well and the balance of the GI tract is seriously disrupted. It should also be noted that many of the situations where antibiotics are prescribed are not based on sound medical reasoning and thorough diagnosis. Diarrhea, constipation, fever, vomiting and other symptoms may not be caused by infection and therefore will not be improved by antibiotics. And, since the immune system in infants is still fragile, it can be permanently derailed.

Dr. Gary Huffnagle, professor at University of Michigan, found through his research that antibiotics knock out bacteria in the gut, allowing fungi to take over temporarily until the bacteria grow back after the antibiotics are stopped. His research indicates that altering intestinal microflora this way can lead to changes in the entire system that may produce symptoms elsewhere.

Too powerful a weapon to fight the intruder... Like using a machine gun to kill an invading rat, antibiotics are far too strong for most uses and, like any other drug, they should be respected and used very sparingly only when completely necessary. All too often, diseases emerging later in life are being linked to early use of antibiotics. Such diseases include Crohn's disease, asthma, allergies and inflammatory bowel diseases (IBS and IBD).

Our increasing dependence on antibiotics for almost any ailment is leading to the destruction of our essential healthy and helpful microflora. Through this abuse we are also creating superbugs, which are pathogens that have evolved or mutated in order to survive the effects of antibiotic treatment. Antibiotics' effectiveness is there-

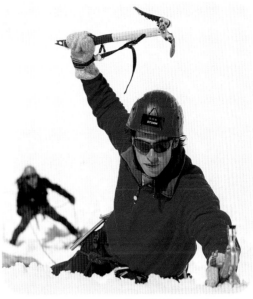

Antibiotics overpower beneficial bacteria and leave lasting effects.

fore waning and doctors are forced to use more expensive and toxic drugs against these superbugs. This is further fueling the problem – like a nuclear power plant reaching critical mass.

Probiotics – Restore Health and Vitality at Any Age

Few of us start out with a good microbial balance within our bodies in today's polluted world and few can maintain that optimal balance without help. Pollution in our air, food and water, and our increased dependency on antibiotics as a cure-all, have increased our chances of contracting a life-threatening disease or debilitating ailment. These contaminants also deplete the naturally occurring microflora, further harming us.

Fight back with a natural fortifier... In addition to taking a proactive approach to help our planet by decreasing pollution, there is a simple solution to the dilemma that will help to return your quality of life. High-quality selected probiotic bacteria strains can restore and maintain your gut microflora, enabling you to have the vital, healthful and happy life you deserve. Probiotics can protect against and aid in fighting many common ailments, such as heartburn, indigestion, lactose intolerance, gastric inflammation, allergies, yeast overgrowth and osteoporosis.

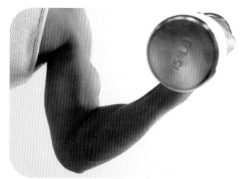

Supplementing with probiotic bacteria strengthens your intestinal microflora and your immune system.

Even global leaders are taking notice. The World Health Organization, in conjunction with the Food and Agricultural Organization of the United Nations, has called together an international committee of scientific experts to promote the benefits of probiotics. The European Commission, in a coordinated approach to improving the health of European citizens, has initiated a human health research program. Scientific and medical research groups from sixteen countries are exploring the relationships between intestinal bacteria and human health and disease, and defining probiotic therapies to be used for infections, chronic disease and healthy aging.

There is so much conflicting information about diet, exercise and nutritional recommendations today that it is no wonder if you are confused. With the overwhelming amount of choices now available on health and supplement store shelves it is also not surprising that you cannot decide what is needed for proper supplementation. It takes research and, perhaps, experimentation to decipher what your particular body needs. However, due to the environment we all share, one choice is clear and universally required. Thousands of articles published in scientific journals report overwhelming evidence about the health effects of selected probiotic strains of bacteria. Supplementing your diet daily with guaranteed super strains is the single most important addition to protect your health. Selected super strains form the barrier against the invading hostile microorganisms that lie in wait to assault your immune system.

Purchasing Probiotics – Choose the Right One

Shopping for probiotic bacteria is similar to shopping for any other important dietary supplement. You want to purchase the best possible product that will always do the best possible job. Unfortunately, I have found in my many years within the industry that far too many manufacturers and suppliers are only interested in making a buck instead of providing consumers with a viable and effective product. However, there are important things you can look for while comparison shopping to ensure you receive your money's worth.

While it's easy to say that a product is of exceptional quality, it is often difficult to monitor these standards. Quality control of any natural ingredients in a supplement is complicated when you consider culturing (growing), manufacturing, packaging, shipping and storage methods.

Buy from companies that stand behind their product. Make sure the manufacturer has International Drug Good Manufacturing Practice (GMP) certification. This recognition is only given to manufacturers that follow pharmaceutical standards in preparation and production of a product. It also ensures that the product has been tested for purity, potency and safety in all stages from the first culturing of the bacteria through to the expiration date. Currently there is only one probiotics manufacturer that has been given this certification.

It is also important to look for a manufacturer that produces only probiotics. With only one focus, the company can concentrate its research, development and improvements to produce the best supplements available. The products will have been created by experts who understand and appreciate beneficial bacteria and specific strain benefits and characteristics. Even more important, the manufacturer will have the capability of producing consistent products, ensuring that you get the same quality each and every time.

May not be actual size

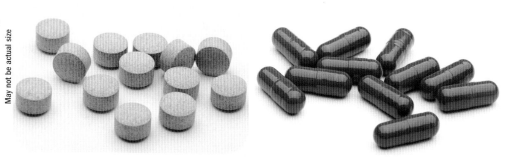

Look for probiotic bacteria products that do not contain artificial colors or flavors.

Packaging promises... Your first and most important step in finding the right probiotic product is to select one that offers a guaranteed potency through a printed expiration date, not the date of manufacture. This will ensure maximum potency at time of consumption. A truthful manufacturer will list the bacterial strains on the label. However, numerous studies have found that the label does not always match the strains found in the product. Be sure that the product you are buying contains only selected super strains with proven health benefits. These strains must be listed on the label. The potency of each type of bacteria should also be declared on the label in colony forming units (scientific measure of living bacteria). Beware of manufacturers that list the bacterial counts in milligrams. I know, governmental agencies know and science dictates that this is a worthless measure of viability. Milligrams are a measure of weight, not potency, so you have no guarantee that the bacteria are alive.

Since probiotic bacteria are extremely light- and moisture-sensitive, only purchase products packaged in dark glass bottles with tin lids. These bottles and lids protect the bacteria from the damaging effects of heat, light or moisture. Plastic is permeable and, therefore, not a suitable packaging material for delicate probiotics. It is also important to purchase probiotics that are shipped and stored under refrigeration to keep the bacteria viable through the expiration date. Beware of products claiming that no refrigeration is necessary. If exposed to even the slightest amount of heat, light or moisture, the bacteria will begin to grow. In a close-ended system, such as a bottle, capsule or wafer (chewable tablet), the bacteria are in an arrested state of growth and a fraction of moisture can stimulate the life cycle. In such an environment the bacteria use up the food source and die. In contrast, your body is an open-ended system where food enters and provides an opportunity for beneficial bacteria to thrive.

Top Tip: Do not buy probiotic supplements containing FOS, fructooligosaccharide, as the effects are uncertain. The second book in the series will include a section on this topic.

The cold hard facts… Though you will notice several types of probiotics on stores' regular, non-refrigerated shelves, these have not been proven effective. There are no heat-stable or shelf-stable probiotic products that have been validated by an independent government agency. In fact, three scientific studies conducted by Bastyr University, Consumer

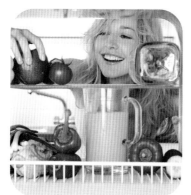

Always make room for your probiotic products.

Labs and *Consumer Reports* revealed continuous failures of products to meet their label declarations. A similar breach of customer trust occurred in Australia, resulting in the recall of 1,600 dietary supplement products. Only a specific type of packaging, refrigerated handling and guaranteed potency through a printed expiration date provide trustworthy assurance of a viable product.

A supplement is only as good as the portion of it that actually gets where it is supposed to go and then gets properly absorbed to benefit your body. Many supplements, particularly probiotics, are ineffective because they don't do these jobs properly. Good bacteria are very delicate and, if not protected, they can be destroyed by corrosive digestive acids long before they are delivered to your intestines.

If you are purchasing a multi-strain product, look for one that is prepared in a very particular type of delivery system for your body. The best type is micro-enrobed in an oil matrix system, which covers the bacteria in a protective bubble. This separates the bacteria, keeping them healthy and strong. The oil matrix protects the bacteria against the onslaught of stomach acid. Once in the small intestines, the bile that is present will break down the oil-matrix barrier and the bacteria will be released. Only selected strains of beneficial bacteria that have been independently tested for bile resistance (i.e. meaning bile will not destroy it), are powerful enough to help you. Be leery of so-called entero-coated supplements. Entero-coating is designed for pharmaceutical products and is not designed to protect probiotic bacteria.

Be sure to purchase a probiotic product with the supernatant intact. This is the culturing medium, such as milk, garbanzo (chickpea), or soy base, used to grow the bacteria. It is full of beneficial byproducts that result from the growing of probiotic bacteria. Not only does it offer many additional beneficial components, it also buffers the bacteria against stomach acid, ensuring that you receive the maximum benefits where they are needed.

Added Benefits – The Importance of the Supernatant

Unique probiotic manufacturers grow their beneficial bacteria in a culturing medium, usually milk or a non-dairy base such as organic garbanzo or organic soy base. As the bacteria grow, they transform the medium into a new substance that is known as the supernatant. This supernatant contains beneficial metabolic byproducts that are helpful to both you and the bacteria themselves. These include vitamins, enzymes, amino acids and antimicrobial compounds such as hydrogen peroxide and acidophilin, which is a specific substance harmful to other bacteria but not the human host. They also include peptides helpful in lowering blood pressure, antioxidants that destroy dangerous free radicals and promote health and longevity, and immuno-stimulants, which jump-start your immune system. Keeping the bacteria and its all-important supernatant together, called full-culture processing, retains this culturing medium and all of its benefits. This process is more expensive but the resulting product is well worth the extra cost because the supernatant increases the benefits of the product by up to fifty percent.

Top Tip: Make sure that the probiotic product you purchase has the supernatant intact in order to obtain the optimal benefits for your money.

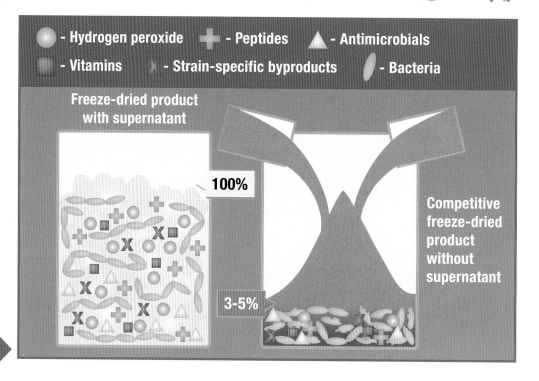

Legend:
- Hydrogen peroxide
- Peptides
- Antimicrobials
- Vitamins
- Strain-specific byproducts
- Bacteria

Freeze-dried product with supernatant

100%

3-5%

Competitive freeze-dried product without supernatant

Higher quality ingredients and processing mean a more effective product. All too often, manufacturers focus on the cost of production and strip the supernatant away from the bacteria using mechanical processes, leaving a mere three to five percent of concentrated bacteria. The bacterial concentrate is then freeze-dried and mixed with inexpensive filler, which composes about ninety-five percent of the supplement, to lower the cost of the product. These cheap fillers do not nourish the bacteria or protect it from the stomach acid, as does the supernatant.

Supernatant super strength... Researchers have demonstrated that many of the beneficial properties of probiotic microorganisms can be attributed to the active enzymes, vitamins, peptides, amino acids, antioxidants and powerful antimicrobial substances the beneficial bacteria have produced in the supernatant. The intrinsic supernatant also has another important function. It is the bacteria supplement's initial means of surviving within the human gut. It functions as a buffer, protecting against exposure to the digestive juices, including hydrochloric acid within the stomach. Studies show that probiotic products retaining their supernatant are remarkably more effective and have a longer guaranteed shelf life. Dr. Rasic, a noted researcher from Novi Sad Institute in Yugoslavia, observed a greatly reduced number of pathogenic bacteria where a

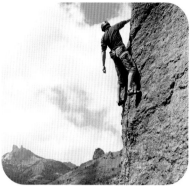

Hang on to optimal health by increasing your levels of beneficial bacteria.

Lactobacillus acidophilus, DDS-1 super strain product contained large numbers of viable acidophilus bacteria and a milk-based supernatant. Numerous research studies underscore the importance of the intrinsic supernatant. A good example of why keeping the supernatant intact is important – bacteria and the intrinsic supernatant are like the natural whole wheat kernel with all its complete goodness (including its bran and germ) before it has been lost by over-processing.

The presence of natural antimicrobial substances in the supernatant along with the high numbers of viable probiotic cells of selected strains have been identified in independent studies as highly effective agents against bad bacteria and yeast including *Escherichia coli* (*E. coli*), *Candida albicans* and *Staphylococcus aureus*. These are only a few of the pathogens that can cause a multitude of illnesses, including food poisoning, diarrhea, chronic fatigue, allergies, heart infections, skin infections, organ failure and even death.

Supernatant springs good bacteria to life… The supernatant provides a natural and ready source of nourishment and protection for the beneficial bacteria while they remain in a state of arrested growth (like sleeping or hibernation) until they are consumed. When ingested, they have an immediate source of food and protection within the supernatant, which enables them to survive once in the body. It is presumed by scientists that the primary and production cultures of the beneficial bacteria are only dormant (when all biological functions actually stop rather than just slow down) when stored in liquid nitrogen. However, finished products only require normal refrigeration.

The Best of the Best – High-Quality Probiotics

Using probiotics to maximize your health will only be effective when you choose premier quality supplements containing proven super strains of beneficial bacteria and their own supernatant. There are only a few products that deliver specific health benefits.

What a supplement *doesn't* include is also important… In addition to products not working the way they are supposed to, there are other considerations. Some have unintentionally added toxic elements. Scientific studies have proven that many inferior probiotic products do not even contain the ingredients listed on the label and, even worse, they contain harmful ingredients. I think it is better to be safe than sorry and reconsider buying lesser priced substitutions because they offer uneven results and failure.

High-quality, select probiotic products contain only super strains that have been proven effective. Seek recommended products that have been validated under International Drug GMP certification for potency, purity, safety, strain identification and stability by independent government agencies, such as the Australian Therapeutic Goods Agency. If you follow my guidelines, you will be able to find the brand names of the products that will provide you with the most health benefits for your money.

Become a judge... Compare categories. There are three levels in my Probiotic Supplementation Program which has been thoroughly researched over the past twenty-five years – GOOD, BETTER, BEST.

Level One – Good

Single strain probiotic bacteria are available as loose powders or as powder product in veggie capsules. One dose of high-quality powdered products contains 2 billion colony forming units

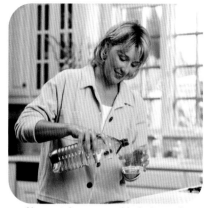

Always take your probiotic bacteria powder or capsules with unchilled, non-chlorinated water or non-acidic juice.

(CFU) per gram. A capsule of high-quality probiotic bacteria contains a dose of 2 billion CFUs per capsule. For added convenience, *Lactobacillus bulgaricus,* LB-51 super strain may come in a chewable dairy-based wafer with a usual dose of 1 billion CFUs per two wafers. There are no known toxic levels of these bacteria strains, so the dose may be increased as desired. Powders should be dissolved using a clean, dry utensil and glass, in eight ounces of unchilled, non-chlorinated water or non-acidic juice (apple or pear). Capsules can also be taken along with a powder regimen (and vice versa) if you wish, for optimal results and desired health benefits. The amounts described are for adults; reduce amounts for children depending on their weight. Always consult your healthcare professional prior to starting a supplement regimen.

> **Top Tip:** Colony forming unit (CFU) – a measure of potency. Vital bacteria cells cluster together in short or long chains as they grow and multiply. Each one is counted as a colony forming unit. CFU is the accepted potency declaration in the Probiotic Quality and Safety Standards read into The Congressional Record in 1994. Be wary of manufacturers measuring in milligrams because this is a measurement of weight only and not a measure of live bacteria.

Super strain bacteria are cultured in a special way on a selected growth medium so that specific health properties can be guaranteed. For example, *Lactobacillus acidophilus,* DDS-1 super strain produces acidophilin when it is grown in milk. However, many people cannot digest milk products and prefer a dairy free product. Through rigorous scientific research and development, other validated super strains (such as *Lactobacillus acidophilus*, NAS strain, *Bifidobacterium bifidum*, Malyoth strain and *Lactobacillus bulgaricus*, LB-51 strain) have been cultured in other growth media, retaining their special properties. The following table lists the choices suggested for selected super strains of probiotic bacteria products.

May not be actual size

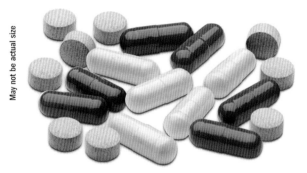

Probiotic supplements are available in powder, wafer and capsule form.

Top Tip: "One size fits all" supplements don't always accurately provide your unique personal requirements. Probiotics supplementation should be developed according to each person's needs in order to maintain optimal health or to regain health. For best results, design your personal supplementation plan by calling a company offering experienced probiotic consultants to guide you in selecting the program to suit your preferences. Probiotic supplementation is so important that investing the time to plan an optimal program will ensure a big payoff in wonderful health benefits.

Probiotic Product Choices to Suit Your Personal Preference

Bacteria Super Strain	Dairy (Single strain bacteria product grown in milk base)	Dairy Free (Single strain bacteria product grown in organic garbanzo or organic soy base)	General Target Areas (Specific conditions in comprehensive table)
L. acidophilus, DDS-1	– Loose Powder – Powder Product in Veggie Capsules	– Loose Powder*	– Small intestine health – Urinary tract health
L. acidophilus, NAS		– Loose Powder – Powder Product in Veggie Capsules	– Small intestine health – Vaginal tract health
B. bifidum, Malyoth	– Loose Powder	– Loose Powder – Powder Product in Veggie Capsules	– Large intestine (colon) health – Supports liver health
L. bulgaricus, LB-51	– Loose Powder – Chewable wafers	– Powder Product in Veggie Capsules	– Scavenger that cleans up the GI tract – Digestive aid
B. infantis, NLS	– Loose Powder+		– Infant GI tract health – Alleviates allergies

Grown in a green vegan formula; +Grown in cow's milk or goat's milk

53

Level Two – Better

When you seek an ultimately potent probiotic supplement, select a three-in-one probiotic oil matrix capsule that delivers three types of super strain bacteria. This will maximize the health of your entire GI system. These three-in-one capsules are available as a dairy free product with a total of 30 billion CFU super strain bacteria in each capsule guaranteed through a printed expiration date. This product covers the entire GI tract, offering the benefits of three powerful strains. Hydrogen peroxide-producing *Lactobacillus acidophilus,* NAS super strain protects the small intestine with demonstrated antimicrobial activity against pathogens, such as *Candida albicans. Bifidobacterium bifidum,* Malyoth super strain is the defender of the large intestine (colon) and a strong supporter of healthy liver function. *Lactobacillus bulgaricus,* LB-51 super strain is a powerful digestive aid that scavenges the entire GI tract to clean it up and supports the function of the other two bacteria.

These dairy free proprietary probiotic oil matrix capsules keep the beneficial bacteria separated and noncompetitive so they don't compete for dominance and destroy each other. This system protects the beneficial bacteria on their journey through your stomach's acidic environment, thus offering maximum benefits to the small and large intestines.

Probiotic Oil Matrix Three-in-one Super Capsule		
Bacteria Super Strain	**Each Capsule Contains:**	**Minimum Adult Dosage**
L. acidophilus, NAS	5 billion CFU	- 1 capsule per day maintenance dose
B. bifidum, Malyoth	20 billion CFU	- May be increased as desired
L. bulgaricus, LB-51	5 billion CFU	- Not toxic at any level

Level Three – Best

You can use "layers" of probiotic supplements to deliver the most powerful health effect. By choosing single strain loose powder products of *Lactobacillus acidophilus,* DDS-1 or NAS strains, *Bifidobacterium bifidum*, Malyoth strain or *Lactobacillus bulgaricus,* LB-51 strain or the same strains of beneficial bacteria products in veggie capsules, you will achieve a concentrated and very particular health benefit that is provided by that unique strain. This may be important if your particular needs or symptoms are focused in one area. For example, if you need immediate digestive relief and also continual digestive support, take two or more chewable dairy wafers of *Lactobacillus bulgaricus,* LB-51 strain. The powerful three-in-one probiotic oil matrix capsules are the simplest way to fortify your immune system, strengthen the super probiotics benefits and reach optimal health in general. You may mix and match bacteria powder products, bacteria powder products in veggie capsules, three-in-one oil matrix capsule products and chewable wafer products to receive your desired results. Here are some suggested examples. You may find these examples suit your needs perfectly or they may need to be adjusted to meet your individual needs.

Top Tip: You will benefit from probiotic bacteria supplements, even if you are unable to manage the entire regimen recommended for a particular condition. It is better to take some than nothing at all. Just like getting benefits from an exercise routine, some exercise is better than none!

Suggested Bacterial Supplement Dosages (Minimum Amount) Found in Select Probiotic Products

Condition ◆	Bacteria Super Strain Used	Loose Powders: Single Strain bacteria grown in milk or organic garbanzo or organic soy base	Powder Products in Veggie Capsules: Single Strain bacteria grown in milk, organic garbanzo or organic soy base	Three-in-one Oil Matrix Capsule & Chewable Dairy Wafer⁺
General Use	L. acidophilus, DDS-1 or NAS B. bifidum, Malyoth L. bulgaricus, LB-51	- $\frac{1}{2}$ tsp or more of each bacterial strain daily	- 1 or more of each bacterial strain capsule daily	- 1 or more capsules daily - 2 or more L. bulgaricus wafers daily as needed
Acid Reflux/Heartburn	L. acidophilus, DDS-1 or NAS B. bifidum, Malyoth L. bulgaricus, LB-51	- 1 tsp or more of each bacterial strain daily before meals	- 2 or more of each bacterial strain capsule daily before meals	- 1 to 3 or more capsules daily - 2 or more L. bulgaricus wafers daily as needed
Acne	L. acidophilus, DDS-1 or NAS B. bifidum, Malyoth L. bulgaricus, LB-51	- $\frac{1}{2}$ tsp of each bacterial strain twice daily	- 1 or more of each bacterial strain capsule twice daily	- 1 or more capsules daily - 2 or more L. bulgaricus wafers daily as needed

Condition	Bacterial Strains			
Allergies	L. acidophilus, DDS-1 or NAS B. bifidum, Malyoth L. bulgaricus, LB-51 B. infantis, NLS* *Cow or goat milk base	- ½ tsp or more of each bacterial strain daily	- 1 or more of each bacterial strain capsule daily along with B. infantis powder	- 1 to 3 capsules daily along with B. infantis powder - 2 or more L. bulgaricus wafers daily as needed
Antibiotics Always take probiotics two hours away from antibiotics	L. acidophilus, DDS-1 or NAS B. bifidum, Malyoth L. bulgaricus, LB-51	- 1 to 2 tsp of each bacterial strain two hours following antibiotics and before bed - 2 to 6 tsp of each bacterial strain daily for two weeks after antibiotic treatment	- 2 to 4 of each bacterial strain capsule two hours following antibiotics and before bed - 4 to 12 of each bacterial strain capsule daily for two weeks after antibiotic treatment	- 3 to 4 capsules daily two hours after antibiotics and before bed - 4 to 6 capsules daily for two weeks after antibiotic treatment - 2 or more L. bulgaricus wafers daily as needed
Candidiasis ♣	L. acidophilus, DDS-1 or NAS B. bifidum, Malyoth L. bulgaricus, LB-51	- ½ tsp of both L. acidophilus and B. bifidum before meals - ¼ tsp of L. bulgaricus after meals	- 1 capsule before meals of both L. acidophilus and B. bifidum - 1 capsule of L. bulgaricus after meals	- 1 or more capsules daily
Cholesterol Assistance	L. acidophilus, DDS-1 or NAS B. bifidum, Malyoth	- ½ tsp of each bacterial strain with meals	- 1 or more of each bacterial strain capsule with meals	- 1 or more capsules daily - 2 or more L. bulgaricus wafers daily as needed

Suggested Bacterial Supplement Dosages (Minimum Amount) Found in Select Probiotic Products

Condition◆	Bacteria Super Strain Used	Loose Powders: Single Strain bacteria grown in milk or organic garbanzo or organic soy base	Powder Products in Veggie Capsules: Single Strain bacteria grown in milk, organic garbanzo or organic soy base	Three-in-one Oil Matrix Capsule & Chewable Dairy Wafer†
Cold Sores	*L. acidophilus*, DDS-1 or NAS *B. bifidum*, Malyoth *L. bulgaricus*, LB-51	- ¹/₂ tsp of each bacterial strain before meals, making sure to swish liquid in mouth	- 1 of each bacterial strain capsule three times daily in addition to powder dose	- 1 or more capsules daily - 2 or more *L. bulgaricus* wafers daily as needed
Constipation	*L. acidophilus*, DDS-1 or NAS *B. bifidum*, Malyoth *L. bulgaricus*, LB-51	- ¹/₂ tsp of each bacterial strain before meals - 2 tsp of *B. bifidum* or *L. bulgaricus* before bedtime	- 1 of each bacterial strain capsule before meals - 4 capsules of *B. bifidum* or *L. bulgaricus* before bed	- 1 or more capsules daily - 2 or more *L. bulgaricus* wafers daily as needed
Crohn's Disease	*L. acidophilus*, DDS-1 or NAS *B. bifidum*, Malyoth *L. bulgaricus*, LB-51	- 2 tsp or more of each bacterial strain three times daily	- 4 or more of each bacterial strain capsule three times daily	- 2 to 4 capsules three times daily - 2 or more *L. bulgaricus* wafers daily as needed
Diarrhea♣	*L. acidophilus*, DDS-1 or NAS *B. bifidum*, Malyoth *L. bulgaricus*, LB-51	- ¹/₂ tsp or more of each bacterial strain every hour until symptoms subside	- 1 or more of each bacterial strain capsule every hour until symptoms subside	- 3 or more capsules daily until symptoms subside - 2 or more *L. bulgaricus* wafers daily as needed

Condition	Strains			
Gas/Bloating	L. acidophilus, DDS-1 or NAS B. bifidum, Malyoth L. bulgaricus, LB-51	- $1/2$ tsp or more of each bacterial strain daily	- 1 or more of each bacterial strain capsule daily	- 1 or more capsules daily - 2 or more L. bulgaricus wafers daily as needed
Infants	B. infantis, NLS* *Cow or goat milk base	- Start at $1/4$ tsp daily; increase gradually		
Insomnia	B. bifidum, Malyoth	- $1 1/2$ tsp or more before bed	- 3 to 4 capsules before bed	- 1 capsule during the day - 2 or more L. bulgaricus wafers daily as needed
Irritable Bowel Syndrome (IBS)	L. acidophilus, DDS-1 or NAS B. bifidum, Malyoth L. bulgaricus, LB-51 B. infantis, NLS* *Cow or goat milk base	- $1/2$ tsp of each bacterial strain daily before meals - 3 tsp once daily or more often as needed	- 1 or more of each bacterial strain capsule daily before meals along with B. infantis powder	- 1 capsule two to three times daily along with B. infantis powder - 2 or more L. bulgaricus wafers daily as needed
Lactose Intolerance	L. acidophilus, DDS-1	- Start at $1/8$ tsp daily; increase gradually to $1/2$ tsp or more	- When powder dose is tolerated, add 1 capsule three times daily following powder dose	- 1 or more capsules daily - 2 or more L. bulgaricus wafers daily as needed

Suggested Bacterial Supplement Dosages (Minimum Amount) Found in Select Probiotic Products

Condition ◆	Bacteria Super Strain Used	Loose Powders: Single Strain bacteria grown in milk or organic garbanzo or organic soy base	Powder Products in Veggie Capsules: Single Strain bacteria grown in milk, organic garbanzo or organic soy base	Three-in-one Oil Matrix Capsule & Chewable Dairy Wafer+
Liver Detoxification	L. acidophilus, DDS-1 or NAS L. bulgaricus, LB-51 B. bifidum, Malyoth	- 1/2 tsp of both L. acidophilus and L. bulgaricus three times daily - 2 tsp of B. bifidum three times daily	- 1 capsule of both L. acidophilus and L. bulgaricus three times daily - 4 capsules of B. bifidum three times daily	- 2 or more capsules three times daily - 2 or more L. bulgaricus wafers daily as needed
Pregnancy/ Nursing	B. infantis, NLS* *Cow or goat milk base L. acidophilus, DDS-1 or NAS B. bifidum, Malyoth L. bulgaricus, LB-51	- 1/2 to 1 tsp daily before meals - 1/2 tsp of each bacterial strain daily before meals	- 1 of each bacterial strain capsule daily before meals along with B. infantis powder	- 1 or more capsules daily along with B. infantis powder - 2 or more L. bulgaricus wafers daily as needed
Ulcerative Colitis	L. acidophilus, DDS-1 or NAS B. bifidum, Malyoth L. bulgaricus, LB-51	- 1/2 to 1 1/2 tsp of each bacterial strain daily	- 1 to 3 of each bacterial strain capsule daily	- 1 capsule three to four times daily - 2 or more L. bulgaricus wafers daily as needed

Condition	Strains			
Urinary Tract Infection	L. acidophilus, DDS-1 or NAS B. bifidum, Malyoth L. bulgaricus, LB-51	- 1 tsp of each bacterial strain twice daily for two weeks	- 2 of each bacterial strain capsule twice daily for two weeks	- 2 or more capsules daily for two weeks - 2 or more L. bulgaricus wafers daily as needed
Vaginitis	L. acidophilus, DDS-1 or NAS B. bifidum, Malyoth L. bulgaricus, LB-51	- 1 tsp of each bacterial strain twice daily for two weeks	- 2 of each bacterial strain capsule twice daily for two weeks	- 2 or more capsules daily for two weeks - 2 or more L. bulgaricus wafers daily as needed
Weight Loss	L. bulgaricus, LB-51	- 1 to 3 tsp or more before meals	- 2 to 6 capsules or more before meals	- 1 capsule three times daily - 2 or more L. bulgaricus wafers daily as needed

◆ The probiotic supplements outlined in this book are not drugs and can be taken safely in larger amounts and greater frequency than recommended. This will not cause an imbalance – i.e. too many good bacteria. High-quality probiotics may cause a die-off of bad bacteria, yeasts and fungi. The probiotics cause large numbers of the bad bugs to leave the body through the regular channels of elimination and toxic waste (through bowels and kidneys). When the toxic die-off is large in number, the kidney and bowel routes of elimination become crowded and unable to accommodate the mass at one time. Known as the Herxheimer Reaction, this toxic die-off can lead to temporary symptoms of headaches, gas and bloating. If this happens to you, don't panic. This is a positive sign that your body is healing by ridding itself of harmful organisms and their toxic byproducts. Just lessen the amount of probiotics you are taking and slowly increase to the desired dose.

+ Wafers sweetened with beet fructose contain only five calories per serving (2 wafers).

❣ Candidiasis: Individuals with Candidiasis (Candida albicans) should limit or avoid products with sugars, including unprocessed and naturally occuring sugars that are found in fruit, honey and maple syrup. See general information below.

◢ Diarrhea: Contact your healthcare professional if diarrhea lasts more than two days or if fever or other symptoms are present, such as abdominal swelling or blood in the stool.

● Some ethnic groups may have severe allergic reactions to milk. Make certain your infant or child does not have a severe milk allergy by checking with your healthcare professional.

General Information: Avoid all products with high fructose corn syrup, artificial sweeteners, chemical additives and excessive processing. Avoid fast foods or prepared foods. Stick to simple or freshly prepared meals. Choose organic meats, poultry, vegetables, fruits, grains, eggs, milk, soy milk, tofu and other food products. Seek dietary regimens that support your particular problem.

Living a Healthy Life – Probiotics and You

A gut feeling… Metchnikoff understood the link between probiotics and longevity. Modern science is finally catching up with his theories. The beneficial bacteria found in probiotics have been used for thousands of years to aid in digestion. Scientific research is now proving that many common and not-so-common ailments are dependent on the function and strength of intestinal bacteria and the efficiency of digestive health. Probiotic supplementation is so important that several nations have empowered their agencies to develop products containing selected single strains of beneficial bacteria for their citizens to consume on a daily basis. No other food or dietary supplement has such a distinction. Probiotic supplements should be taken daily to combat illness and replenish diminishing microflora, which leads to disease.

How do you know if your probiotics are working? Health isn't related as much to the quantity of nutrients you take in as to the amount that actively reaches your organs and is available for your body to assimilate effectively. If you have been taking probiotics regularly you naturally assume and trust that they are doing their job. However, many manufacturers mislead consumers and produce products that do not deliver any health benefits at all. These supplements aren't providing live bacteria and are therefore useless, simply passing through the system as "expensive urine." If you have chosen the right probiotics, you can tell that they're working by the following reactions: You will quickly see that your digestive problems are relieved, bowel elimination will be improved, you will have more energy, you will be less susceptible to colds and flu, and your skin will look brighter and healthier. High-quality probiotics from a reputable manufacturer can assure optimal daily health.

Probiotic supplementation should become a daily ritual just as routine as brushing your teeth.

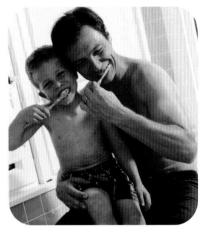

Top Tip: Always choose probiotics from the *Lactobacillus* and *Bifidobacterium* genera (families). Hundreds of scientific articles have been submitted to the Food and Drug Administration to attest the safety of these bacteria at any level of use.

The information provided in this book is meant to help you make an educated choice in your journey to better health. The best form of health insurance is the one provided by nature. Natural beneficial bacteria are the only way to keep your GI tract and immune system healthy, active and working on your behalf. These bacteria are your first line of defense against potentially lethal infections.

It isn't enough to offer better health products...I believe that natural health companies must provide answers. As society begins to question whether mass produced and poorly regulated supplements and medications are indeed all-encompassing cure-alls, it becomes clear that modern science needs to create a new model for human healing. Health should not be based on averages, generalities and covering symptoms, but on natural (in its most complete form) individualized nutrition and remedies that are proven beyond a doubt to work, without side effects. I feel that we must look beyond the obvious variables and symptoms to produce lasting, rather than quick fix solutions, to alleviate health challenges, to provide greater energy and ensure a longer, more fulfilling life.

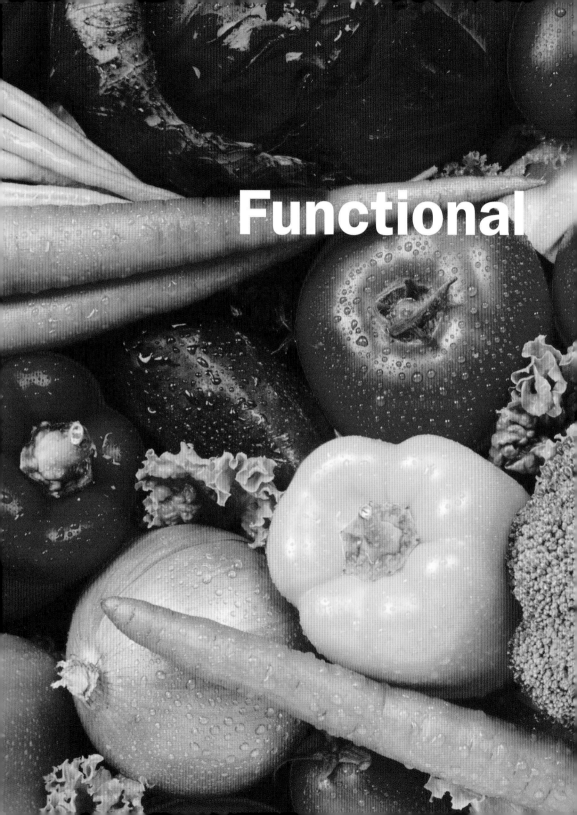

Functional

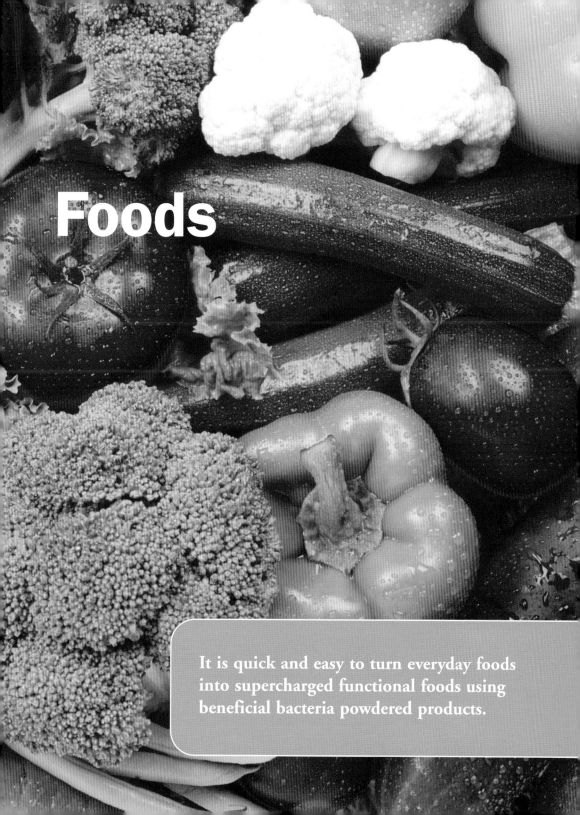

Foods

It is quick and easy to turn everyday foods into supercharged functional foods using beneficial bacteria powdered products.

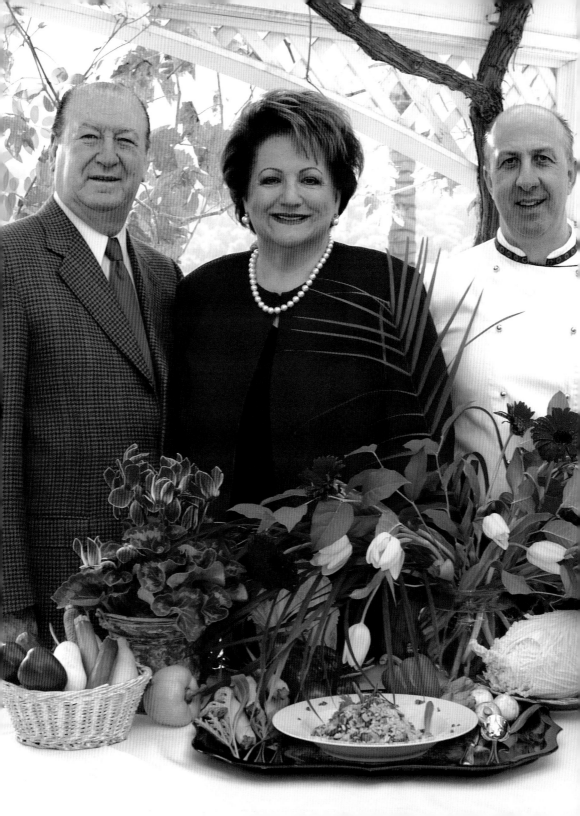

Healthful Habits – Finding Good Health Through Functional Foods

Elie Metchnikoff's observation of the Bulgarians' ability to live a long and healthy life led him to hypothesize about the beneficial properties of yogurt. The probiotic bacteria he found in the yogurt aided in the Bulgarians' health and vitality. Since then, yogurt has been considered a functional food. A functional food offers more health benefits than nourishment alone, meaning that it works like a completely natural medicine with powerful healing properties. Some functional foods, such as kale, spinach and other dark leafy greens, have proven disease-fighting characteristics that work independently, without requiring other foods to assist them. Others become functional by adding a measured sprinkle of selected probiotic powders prior to consumption to increase their healing benefits.

There are many prepared functional foods such as yogurt, kefir and sauerkraut on the market today. All too often, however, the non-beneficial probiotic strains that have been added to the food are based on the relationship (and natural reactions that it brings) between the food and the bacteria, not on the relationship between the bacteria and your health. These foods do not deliver the specific health benefits that can only come from selected super strains of beneficial bacteria.

In order to achieve these specific benefits, simply add selected super strain probiotic powders (containing both the bacteria and the supernatant) to the food. Immediately before consumption, sprinkle 3 to 4 teaspoons of selected beneficial bacteria powder into the food and stir by hand. Follow specific suggested doses to achieve optimal results. Certified organic food products are always

Left: Yordan Trenev, Natasha Trenev and Chef Roberto Carboni show how easy it is to prepare a tasty meal of functional foods with powdered probiotics.

preferred when available. Personal and kitchen hygiene are essential to good health. **Never use wet, damp or dirty utensils when handling probiotic powders.**

When probiotics are added to the following foods, your health will benefit:

• Smoothies and protein shakes
• Infant formula and infant foods (use only *Bifidobacterium infantis* supplements)
• Cereals and grains – Cream of Wheat, kashi, risotto, cornflakes, quinoa, spelt, amaranth, bulgur wheat, couscous, brown or unbleached white rice
• Yogurt, cottage cheese, kefir, liquid yogurt, cream cheese, spreads and butter
• Fruit purees – apple, banana, white peach, papaya and mango
• Salads – green, pasta, potato and tuna
• Juices – grape, guava, non-acidic juices such as apple and pear
• Drinks – soy, rice, almond and dairy milks
• Steamed vegetables and mashed potatoes
• Desserts – ice cream, puddings such as rice pudding, frozen yogurt and confectionery (without high fructose corn syrup, or other detrimental sugars, sweeteners or chemical food agents). These desserts are best when homemade using natural, organically certified ingredients.

When sweeteners are needed, use date sugar, agave syrup, maple syrup, stevia, xylitol or raw, organic sugars.

Follow these specific "dos and don'ts" when preparing food using probiotic bacteria… Food should be tepid, not hot or over 120° F (so as not to kill the live bacteria). Do not add any acidic ingredients, such as vinegar, tomatoes, orange juice, lemons or lemon juice, before or after you add the probiotics. Do not cook food once you have fortified it with the probiotic powder supplement. Consume all food once it has been fortified, ensuring no leftovers are kept.

So-called "predigested" protein powders available on the market are supposed to aid in easy digestion. Please note, these powders are only predigested, at the most, up to five to ten percent. The majority of the digestion of the protein must take place in your system. Depending on the source of the protein powder (such as whey, soy or hemp), you will not experience an efficient breakdown of the protein into its essential components of peptides and amino acids (building blocks of the body's cells) without the selected probiotics to aid digestion.

If you are on a weight loss program, I suggest adding 3 teaspoons of the dairy-based *Lactobacillus bulgaricus,* LB-51 powder to a smoothie or protein shake. I also suggest a three-in-one oil matrix probiotic capsule each day. For optimal results, take 3 teaspoons of the powder three times daily before or with meals. (The second book in this series will include a section on obesity and probiotic bacteria's role in helping weight loss in addition to dealing with specific diseases.)

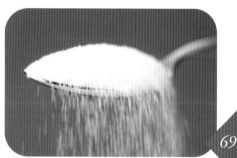

Bifidobacterium infantis is an essential part of a healthy infant's intestinal microflora and life-long health.

As discussed earlier, your infant also needs beneficial bacteria. *Bifidobacterium infantis* is an important part of every infant's diet. It can be added to pumped breast milk or infant formula. Mix $1/4$ to $1/2$ teaspoon of *Bifidobacterium infantis* powder with a small amount of the liquid and stir thoroughly to dissolve. Put the mixture into a bottle and add more breast milk or formula. Shake well to mix. Make certain small or large lumps of probiotic powder are not left behind as this is where the bacteria are found. If you find lumps, gently crush them into the solution. You can also stir $1/4$ to $1/2$ teaspoon of *Bifidobacterium infantis* powder into pureed vegetables, non-acidic fruit (apples, pears and peaches), meat or chicken.

Preparing food with the addition of selected probiotics is easy…
I have chosen some of my favorite quick recipes to share with you and help you get started. As a busy working woman and a devoted mother and wife, I understand the time constraints experienced in today's bustling world and have found that the marketplace can offer many timesaving solutions to a healthy meal. Supermarket shelves are now lined with boxed and prepared foods that are produced specifically for the health conscious. These products are usually organic, containing non-chemical ingredients. I have incorporated these ingredients as a way to show you how quick and easy healthy eating can be. Enjoy good food, good health and long lasting vitality by using natural whole fresh food ingredients and adding beneficial bacteria supplements to any meal. The following are a few suggestions for probiotic enhancement to foods.

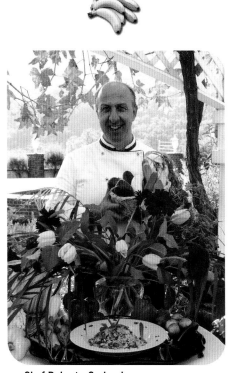

Chef Roberto Carboni

Super Smoothies or Protein Powder Drinks

One of the most popular ways to get a fast, simple and nourishing liquid meal is a smoothie. It can be created from a combination of any non-acidic fruit, non-acidic juice, soy milk, cow's milk, goat's milk, rice milk or yogurt with or without protein powder. Smoothies are prepared using a blender. To turn these yummy drinks into a functional food, first blend all ingredients as you normally would. Make sure to use only non-acidic fruit and fruit juice. In the glass, add 1 1/2 to 3 teaspoons of the probiotic powder (usually 1/2 to 1 teaspoon of each selected powdered probiotic bacteria or any combination of the powdered bacteria product that you desire) and then add 2 to 3 ounces of the blended liquid. Stir until the powder and drink are well mixed. Slowly add the remaining liquid, stirring at all times. Make sure you drink the entire smoothie at one time, not letting it sit. Continually stir if anything settles.

The added effort is minimal compared to the level of improved nourishment you have imparted into your drink. You have increased the digestibility and the ability of your body to absorb all the micronutrients. You will feel full and satisfied without experiencing heaviness in your stomach.

Blueberry Yogurt Smoothie

(Makes 3 servings)

Ingredients
2 cups (1 pint) fresh blueberries or slightly thawed frozen blueberries
1 cup pineapple juice*
8 oz. plain whole or low fat yogurt
Sweetener if desired

Place all ingredients in a blender. Blend until smooth, about 1 minute.
Mix with probiotic powder as described above. Garnish with skewered
blueberries and pineapple. Serve immediately.

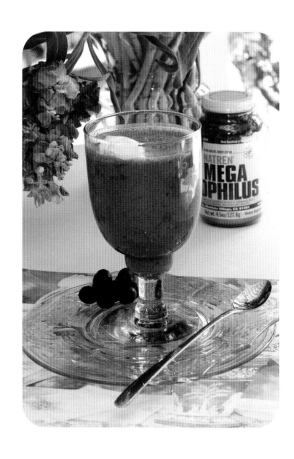

Tropical Silken Tofu Smoothie

(Makes 4 servings)

Ingredients
$^1/_2$ cup silken tofu
1 cup pineapple juice*
1 ripe banana
$^1/_2$ cup crushed pineapple

Place all ingredients in a blender. Blend until smooth, about 1 minute.
Mix with probiotic powder as previously described. Serve immediately.

* This amount of pineapple juice is not too acidic for the probiotic powder product.

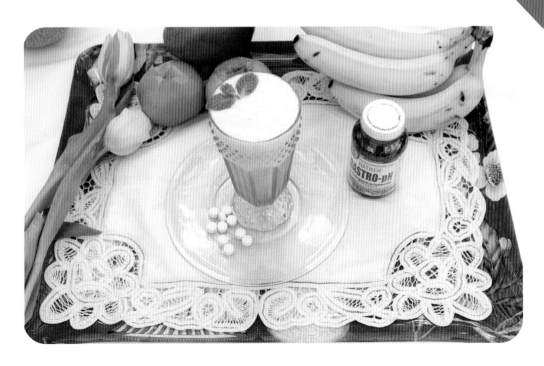

Champion Cereals and Glorious Grains

When you are preparing a cereal or grain dish that has a finished temperature of 120° F or less (higher will destroy good bacteria if it's added), add probiotic powder to increase its nourishing goodness. Sprinkle $1^1/_2$ to 3 teaspoons of the probiotic powder (usually $^1/_2$ to 1 teaspoon of each selected powdered probiotic bacteria product or any combination of the powdered bacteria that you desire). Sprinkle powder onto dish and gently stir in until mixed thoroughly. Use smooth cereals such as oatmeal, Cream of Wheat or grain dishes such as brown rice, lentils, beans, couscous or quinoa. Choose organic, natural products whenever possible. Best results are achieved by adding probiotic bacteria powder to individual servings. Remember to finish the entire dish once it has been fortified with the powder.

Bulgur Wheat for Breakfast

Bulgur is a completely natural, nutritious and versatile wheat with a pleasant flavor.
(Makes 2 servings)

Ingredients
$^1/_2$ cup bulgur wheat
$1^1/_2$ cup water
$^1/_4$ tsp salt (optional)

Microwave
Place ingredients in microwave-safe bowl and microwave on high for 12 to 14 minutes.

I am not in favor in microwaving any food or liquid, including water. I offer this option to people who are not of the same opinion.

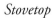

Stovetop
Add bulgur wheat to water and bring to a boil, stirring constantly. Reduce heat, cover and simmer for 10 to 12 minutes or until desired consistency.

Serving Suggestions
Serve bulgur wheat with fruit, nuts or raisins, milk, soy milk or yogurt. Sweeten using honey or any of the sweeteners suggested earlier on page 68.

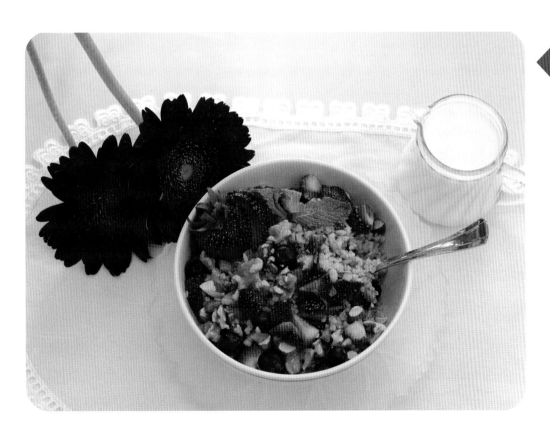

Risotto Di Stagiono

Risotto with baby artichokes, zucchini, mushrooms and cherry tomatoes. (Makes 8 servings)

Ingredients
4 Tbsp extra virgin olive oil
3 cups Arborio rice
$^1/_2$ lb baby artichokes, cleaned
8 cups chicken or vegetable stock, warmed
1 cup dry white wine (optional)
$^1/_2$ lb zucchini, sliced
$^1/_2$ lb cherry tomatoes, quartered
$^1/_2$ lb mushrooms
2 Tbsp grated parmigiono-reggiano cheese
Salt to taste (avoid pepper)
Parsley as desired

In a sauté pan, or risotto pan, warm the olive oil over medium heat. Add the rice and sauté, stirring constantly until the rice is translucent, 3 to 4 minutes. Add the artichokes and stir. Add $^1/_2$ cup of the stock and cook, stirring constantly until it has all been absorbed. Continue adding the stock and wine, if desired, $^1/_2$ cup at a time and zucchini while stirring constantly for another 5 minutes. Add the cherry tomatoes while stirring con-

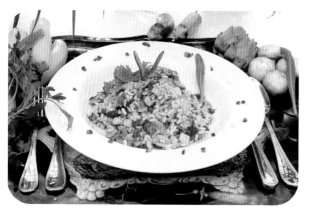

stantly for another 5 minutes. Add the mushrooms and cook until the rice is tender but firm to the bite, about 15 minutes. Stir in the parmigiono-reggiano cheese, salt and parsley. Divide into bowls and enjoy. Do not add the probiotic powder product until food is warm, not hot.

Quinoa Risotto with Arugula and Parmesan

Quinoa, native to Peru, is much like wheat with a subtle nutty flavor.
To prepare this dish as the main course, double the portions.
(Makes 6 servings)

Ingredients
1 Tbsp olive oil
$^1/_2$ yellow onion, chopped
1 clove garlic, minced
1 cup (6 oz) quinoa, well rinsed
$2^1/_4$ cups (18 fl oz) chicken stock, vegetable stock or broth
2 cups (3 oz) chopped, stemmed arugula
1 small carrot, peeled and finely shredded
$^1/_2$ cup ($1^1/_2$ oz) thinly sliced fresh shitake mushrooms
$^1/_4$ cup (1 oz) grated parmesan cheese
$^1/_2$ tsp salt (avoid pepper)

In a large saucepan, heat the olive oil over medium heat. Add the
onion and sauté until soft and translucent, about 4 minutes. Add the
garlic and quinoa and cook for about 1 minute, stirring occasionally to
make sure the garlic does not brown. Add the stock and bring to a boil.
Reduce the heat to low and simmer until the quinoa is almost tender
to the bite but slightly firm in the center, about 12 minutes. The mixture
will be brothy. Stir in the arugula, carrot and mushrooms and simmer
until the quinoa grains have turned from white to translucent, about
2 minutes longer.

Stir in the cheese and season with a small amount of salt. Serve
immediately. Do not add the probiotic bacteria powder until food is
warm, not hot.

Taboule Salad

Whole-wheat couscous or regular couscous is a great replacement for pasta, rice or potatoes.
(Makes 5 servings)

Ingredients
$^1/_2$ cup water
$1^1/_4$ cup dry couscous
$^1/_3$ cup of lemon juice*
6 Tbsp olive oil
1 diced tomato*
$^1/_2$ green pepper, diced
$^1/_2$ onion, chopped
4 Tbsp parsley
1 Tbsp mint
Salt to taste (small amounts of salt)

Boil water and mix with couscous. Add lemon juice and olive oil and stir well. Cover and let sit for 5 minutes. Fluff with a fork. Add tomatoes, green peppers, onion, parsley and mint. Salt to taste and toss lightly. Refrigerate for 15 minutes. Fluff with a fork and add the probiotic powder bacteria immediately prior to serving.

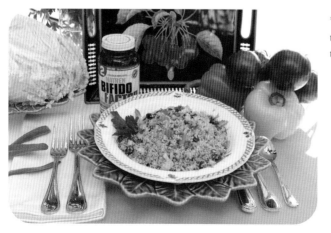

* This amount of citrus and tomatoes within the recipe will not affect the probiotics.

Tasty Treats

Enjoy your cottage cheese, puddings, ice cream, tofu dishes and desserts even more. Sprinkle 1$\frac{1}{2}$ to 3 teaspoons of the probiotic powder (usually $\frac{1}{2}$ to 1 teaspoon of each selected powdered probiotic bacteria or any combination of the powdered bacteria that you desire) on cottage cheese or puddings and mix in. Sprinkle the powders on top of frozen desserts. Make certain that no probiotic powder remains in the melted portion of the dessert on the side of the dish.

Functional Food Facts

Probiotic bacteria powder can be sprinkled over most foods that are not hot, do not have an acidic base and do not contain large amounts of garlic, onions, vinegar, lemon or other acidic byproducts. Avoid white or black pepper, cinnamon or other spices or herbs with antibacterial properties. Go easy on the salt as it is an antibacterial substance. Mixing powdered probiotic bacteria with ingredients that are not recommended means you will lose some or most of the probiotic effect.

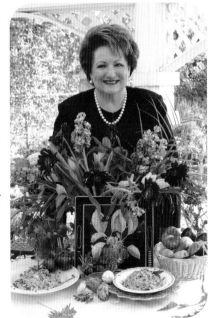

Remember that it is best to take your probiotic bacteria powders or capsules daily following my suggestions. The scientific evidence is in and it overwhelmingly points to the daily use of selected probiotic strains of beneficial bacteria to help fight disease and maximize your health.

Glossary

A

Allergic Rhinitis: An inflammatory nasal response to an allergen. Often includes congestion, sneezing and an itchy or runny nose.

Amino acids: An essential component of protein molecules and necessary building blocks in the body's cellular structure.

Antibiotics: A substance that kills or inhibits the growth of living microorganisms, especially good and bad bacteria found in the gastrointestinal tract. Drugs include penicillin, vancomycin and tetracycline. Natural antibiotics produced by selected strains of beneficial bacteria include bifidin, acidolin, acidophilin, lactolin, lactobacillin, bulgarican and nisin. *Lactobacillus acidophilus,* DDS-1 produces acidophilin only when cultured in milk. Natural antibiotics produced by beneficial bacteria do not damage the body's cellular structure.

Antifungal: A substance that destroys or inhibits the growth of fungi in the body, damaging the liver and other organs at the same time. Drugs include nystatin, ketoconazole and amphotericin. Hydrogen peroxide, a natural antifungal compound produced by selected strains of beneficial bacteria, does not have the toxic side effects of drugs. It is produced in microns and targets only the offending bacteria, thereby not damaging the body's cellular structure.

Antimicrobial: A substance that is capable of destroying or inhibiting the growth of a range of microorganisms, such as bacteria, fungi or viruses. Antimicrobials produced by selected strains of beneficial bacteria include natural antibiotics, bacteriocins, hydrogen peroxide, lactic acid, acetic acid and formic acid. Production is strain specific and induced by specialized production methods.

Antioxidant: A substance that protects body cells from the damaging effects of oxidation (an oxygen process), which includes deterioration of body cells and organs, environmental damage and the aging process.

Atherosclerosis: The deposition of plaque containing cholesterol and fat-soluble materials on the innermost layer of the walls of large and medium-sized arteries. Expansion of the plaque deposit restricts blood flow and increases the risk of coronary artery disease and stroke. High cholesterol levels and inflammation are often present. Selected strains of beneficial bacteria have been found to lower blood and liver total cholesterol levels and reduce inflammation.

Atopic Disease: A common allergy that occurs in specific areas of the body, e.g. hay fever, asthma, eczema. Selected strains of beneficial bacteria assist in allergy management by boosting immune function and by calming down the exaggerated response toward a foreign agent when the immune system over-reacts.

B

Bacteria: Single-celled microorganisms that can either be friendly or cause disease. Selected strains of beneficial bacteria are normally present in a healthy body and protect it from invading organisms.

Bacteriocins: A natural antimicrobial substance produced by certain selected strains of bacteria and harmful to other strains of bacteria, e.g. beneficial bacteria produce acidocin, plantaricin and lactococcin bacteriocins, which inhibit pathogens such as the food-poisoning bacteria, *Bacillus cereus* (soil bacteria) and *Staphylococcus aureus* (found on skin).

Bile: A thick alkaline fluid secreted by the liver and stored in the gallbladder. It is released into the small intestines and helps break down fats and stimulate peristalsis. Selected strains of beneficial bacteria also stimulate peristalsis and regular elimination by the production of lactic, acetic and formic acids.

C

Cirrhotic: A state of inflammation and disease of an organ, particularly the liver. Selected strains of beneficial bacteria, particularly bifidobacteria, reduce the levels of toxins by assisting to excrete them through feces, thereby supporting healthy liver function.

Colonics: A therapy in which the colon is filled with water and flushed out several times to cleanse the colon of waste material and toxins. This also flushes out the beneficial bacteria, leaving the colon vulnerable to domination by hostile bacteria.

Colony Forming Unit (CFU): Colony forming unit is a measure of potency accepted worldwide by scientists and microbiologists. Vital bacteria cells cluster together in short or long chains as they grow and multiply, each one counted as a colony forming unit. CFU is the accepted potency declaration in the Probiotic Quality and Safety Standards read into The Congressional Record in 1994.

E

Entero-coated: Coated in a substance that prevents the release of the contents until after passing through the stomach into the intestine. This process was originally developed for pharmaceutical and over-the-counter (OTC) drugs.

Epithelial cells: Cells that line the digestive tract. They rest on a membrane, which separates the cells from underlying connective tissue. Epithelial cells are protected by layers of selected strains of beneficial bacteria. Without this defense, pathogens and their toxins attack the cells and ultimately build pathways to enter the bloodstream.

Evolutionary medicine: The use of principles of evolution to understand disease processes and design effective medical treatments.

F

Family: A classification of related organisms ranking above a genus. A family usually consists of several genera.

Fermentation: A process in which an agent or live organism causes a complex substance to break down into simpler substances, e.g. the fermentation action of yeast on sugar produces alcohol. The fermentation of proteins, carbohydrates and sugars turns milk into yogurt. Selected strains of beneficial bacteria ferment sugars and the end products include lactic acid, acetic acid and hydrogen peroxide.

Fungi: A diverse group of microorganisms that can exist in more than one form. Fungi have properties that distinguish them from plants so they are placed in their own kingdom, Fungi. Yeasts and molds are major subdivisions of Fungi. The mold state is the pathogenic, aggressive transformed state of the yeast.

G

Gastrointestinal (GI) Tract: The long passageway that starts at the mouth and ends at the anus. It includes the stomach, small intestine and large intestine (colon). The GI tract is home to one hundred trillion bacteria microorganisms that influence the body's health through the digestive and immune functions. Good health depends on beneficial bacteria dominating the harmful bacteria.

Genera (pl. of genus): A category used to classify living things such as plants, animals, bacteria and viruses. A genus consists of two or more closely related, similar species. In *Lactobacillus acidophilus*, the genus is *Lactobacillus*. The species is *acidophilus* and the strain is DDS-1 or NAS.

H

Hyper-Allergenic: The body's exaggerated response to a foreign agent. This auto-immune response can cause inflammation, redness, swelling and pain. Selected strains of beneficial bacteria calm the over-reaction of the immune system and reduce the inflammatory cycle.

I

Inflammation: A defense response by the body to a tissue injury, irritation or infection. The four signs of inflammation are redness (from blood accumulation), warmth (from the heat of the blood), swelling (from the accumulation of fluid) and pain (from injury to the local nerves). Inflammation is the common link and early warning signal of multiple chronic ailments and fatal diseases.

Intrinsic: Essential to and incorporated within the process or product. Not added to or contaminated by the addition of non-essential components.

L

Lactic acid bacteria: A group of non-spore forming bacteria that carry out fermentation of sugars. *Lactobacillus* and *Bifidobacteria* species are lactic acid bacteria.

Lactose: A sugar present in milk. Some people lack sufficient levels of the enzyme lactase, which is needed to digest lactose. These people experience lactose intolerance, which can include cramping, constipation, bloating and diarrhea.

Leaky gut: A common problem when large spaces develop between the epithelial cells of the gut wall and bacteria, toxins or food leak out into the bloodstream and travel to other organs in the body.

M

Macrophage: A scavenger cell found in connective tissue and many body organs. A component of the immune system, they remove some bacteria and foreign bodies by engulfing them from blood and other tissue. Unfortunately, they also play a role in disease. Macrophages can be infected by Human

Immunodeficiency Virus (HIV) and provide a reservoir for virus growth throughout the body.

Metabolic: Relating to the total of all the biochemical processes taking place in living cells.

Micro-enrobe: A process in which the individual bacteria are coated in an oil bubble for protection against corrosive stomach acid.

Microorganism: Any organism too small to be seen with the naked eye, e.g. bacteria, fungi and viruses. These organisms usually need to be magnified five hundred times to be seen.

Mold: An opportunistic form of fungi and yeast, which grows as long, tangled strands of cells. Selected strains of beneficial bacteria inhibit mold and the toxins produced by mold.

O

Oil Matrix: A unique proprietary process in which the bacteria are coated in an oil bubble for protection against corrosive stomach acid, keeping them separated and noncompetitive with one another.

P

Pathogen: A microorganism that produces disease and illness; e.g. *Staphylococcus aureus* and *Escherichia coli* (*E. coli*) cause severe food poisoning and intestinal disease. *Lactobacillus acidophilus*, DDS-1, when grown in milk, has proven antimicrobial activity against these and other harmful microorganisms.

Peristalsis: The rhythmic, wavelike muscular activity of the intestines that helps move along digested food and promotes regular bowel elimination. Selected strains of beneficial bacteria produce lactic, acetic and formic acids that stimulate peristalsis.

Permeable: Able to be penetrated by gases or liquids.

Peptide: A compound composed of two or more amino acids, which are essential building blocks of cellular structure.

Phagocytes: Part of the immune system. A cell able to ingest bacteria, foreign particles and other cells. Phagocytes are divided into two general classes.

1) Microphages are able to ingest bacteria; 2) Macrophages are scavengers that ingest dead tissue and degenerate cells.

Potency: The strength of a substance and its ingredients to work effectively. In this case, it refers to the number of live organisms, measured in colony forming units (CFU). This is the standard scientific unit of measurement for live microorganisms recognized worldwide.

S

Soil Bacteria: Single-celled organisms that live in the soil, e.g. various species of *Bacillus*. Soil bacteria can assume different shapes and are almost indestructible when they form spores. Their safety for use in humans is questionable as they have the ability to transfer antibiotic resistance and are implicated in infections and disease. Some probiotic products for human consumption contain HSOs or soil organisms, which are not recommended.

Species: The smallest unit of classification, ranking below a genus and consisting of a group of microorganisms that have overall similarity but are significantly different from other species, e.g. in *Lactobacillus acidophilus*, NAS, the species is *acidophilus* and the strain is NAS.

Spore: A dormant or resting state of microorganisms. In this state of suspended animation, soil bacteria spores are virtually indestructible when subjected to temperature, pressure or antibiotics.

Strain: A group of organisms of the same species, having distinctive characteristics but not usually considered a separate breed or variety, e.g. in *Lactobacillus acidophilus*, NAS, the strain is NAS.

Supernatant: The growth base for bacteria that contains beneficial metabolic byproducts, including antimicrobial compounds (such as hydrogen peroxide and acidophilin), vitamins, enzymes, cellular building blocks, antioxidants and immunostimulants. Research proves that selected strains of beneficial bacteria retaining their supernatant increase their benefits to the host.

T

T-cells: A component of the immune system, these cells defend against tumor cells and pathogenic organisms inside body cells. These cells can be infected by the Human Immunodeficiency Virus (HIV).

V

Vaginitis: Inflammation of the vagina, often caused by bacterial, viral or fungal infections with *Candida albicans.* Hydrogen peroxide producing *Lactobacillus acidophilus*, NAS has been proven to reduce the incidence of vaginitis caused by *Candida albicans.*

W

Wafers: Chewable tablets, containing *L. Bulgaricus*, LB-51: commonly used for digestive relief. Not just any wafer offers relief.

Y

Yeast: Any single-celled, usually rounded fungi that reproduce by budding. This is the benign form of fungi. Selected strains of beneficial bacteria produce hydrogen peroxide, which inhibits the growth of yeast organisms and mold, another opportunistic form of yeast. Both yeast and mold are dimorphic organisms, meaning that the harmless yeast can turn into a pathogenic mold under the correct conditions.

INDEX

Selected References

Fuller, R., et. al. "Probiotics, the Scientific Basis." Chapman and Hall. New York; 1992.

Madigan, M., Martinko, J. and Parker, J. "Biology of Microorganisms." Prentice Hall. New Jersey; 2003.

Rasic, J. Lj. and Kurmann, J. "Yoghurt." Technical Dairy Publishing House. Denmark; 1978.

Rasic, J. Lj. and Kurmann, J. "Bifidobacteria and Their Role." Birkhauser Verlag. Switzerland; 1983.

Salminen S. and von Wright, A. "Lactic Acid Bacteria." Marcel Dekker, Inc. New York; 1998.

Shortt, C. and O'Brien, J. "Handbook of Functional Dairy Products." CRC Press. New York; 2004.

Tannock, Gerald, et. al. "Probiotics, A Critical Review." Horizon Scientific Press. New Zealand; 1999.

Tierno, Philip M. Jr. "The Secret Life of Germs." Pocket Books, Simon and Schuster. New York; 2001.

Complete citations will be available in scholarly book.